SOD
SEVENTY!
THE GUIDE TO LIVING WELL

Age UK wants everyone to 'love later life' and this highly readable book, which draws on the latest science, helps plot the course for how we can achieve it. Decline is not inevitable but the older we get, the greater the need for positive action if we're to stay fit and well. *Sod Seventy!* explains the how as well as the why of this and as such this book deserves to be essential reading.'

Age UK, 2014

SOD
SEVENTY!

THE GUIDE TO LIVING WELL

MUIR GRAY

illustrated by David Mostyn

BLOOMSBURY
LONDON · NEW DELHI · NEW YORK · SYDNEY

Bloomsbury Sport
An imprint of Bloomsbury Publishing Plc

50 Bedford Square
London
WC1B 3DP
UK

1385 Broadway
New York
NY 10018
USA

www.bloomsbury.com

BLOOMSBURY and the Diana logo are trademarks of Bloomsbury Publishing Plc

First published 2015

© Muir Gray, 2015
Illustrations © David Mostyn, 2015

Muir Gray has asserted his right under the Copyright, Designs and Patents Act, 1988,
to be identified as Author of this work.

British Library Cataloguing-in-Publication Data
A catalogue record for this book is available from the British Library.

Library of Congress Cataloguing-in-Publication data has been applied for.

ISBN: HB: 978-1-4729-1897-0
ePDF: 978-1-4729-1899-4
ePub: 978-1-4729-1898-7

4 6 8 10 9 7 5

Typeset in FS Me by seagulls.net

Printed and bound in Great Britain by CPI Group (UK) Ltd, Croydon CR0 4YY

MIX
Paper from
responsible sources
FSC® C020471

Bloomsbury Publishing Plc makes every effort to ensure that the papers used in the manufacture of our books are natural, recyclable products made from wood grown in well-managed forests. Our manufacturing processes conform to the environmental regulations of the country of origin.

To find out more about our authors and books visit www.bloomsbury.com. Here you will find extracts, author interviews, details of forthcoming events and the option to sign up for our newsletters.

CONTENTS

ACKNOWLEDGEMENTS

I would like to thank the following people who helped improve the content of this book. A number of clinicians commented on the content but full responsibility rests with me. Simon Costain, Guy Duckworth, Diane Stevens, Sally Hope, Claire Parker, Bernard Prendergast, and Howard Williams were the experienced clinicians.

In the publishing team Jackie Rosenthal, John Churchill, Sarah Cole, and Charlotte Croft created a coherent whole with style from the fragments of text the author produced.

Rosemary Lees and Sarah Moore provided excellent support, as always, and the wonderful artist David Mostyn was never stumped, transforming vague ideas into vibrant illustrations with incredible speed.

FOREWORD

The message of this book is that prevention is as relevant at seventy years old as at twenty. We now know that we can postpone many problems that we have assumed to be due to ageing but which well-designed research now proves to be due to loss of fitness, preventable disease and loss of morale. Your health in older age can be improved and this book gives you the recipe for good health in your seventies, and better health in the decades to follow.

Professor Dame Sally Davies
Chief Medical Officer for England

1

AGEING IS NOT A PROBLEM

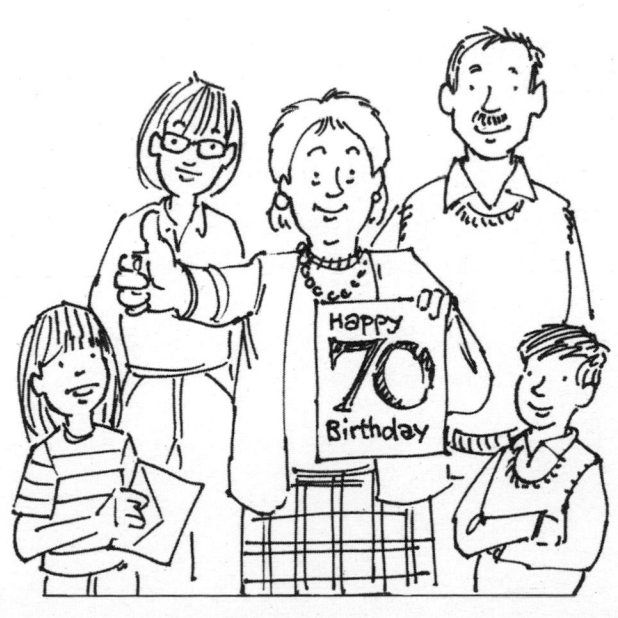

Age is just a number

'Ageing', 'growing old', becoming a 'senior citizen' or a 'retiree' – all these terms are commonly used but mean different things to different people. Some people simply define others as being 'old' if they are older than they are, whether they are 20 or 80!

So let's not get lost in the debate about what these terms mean and whether or not you like to be called 'old', a 'senior citizen', an OAP or an elder. If you are reading this book, you are probably 70 or older. Your age, in numbers, cannot be denied, but your seventieth birthday, or any birthday in your seventies, should not be a cause for gloom. It is a cause for celebration and for taking action to cope with what cannot be denied – namely the effects of the ageing process, which has in fact been working away since you were 30. However, ageing is not the cause of problems in your seventies unless you think it is in control of your health and wellbeing. You can seize control by:

- reducing your risk of developing disease

- becoming fitter, even if you already have one, or more, long term conditions

- adopting a positive attitude to life, its problems and opportunities.

This book is designed to help you achieve all three of these goals.

I recently attended the one hundredth birthday party of a friend. The 'birthday boy' gave a wonderful speech saying, among other things, that a few months earlier he had flown for the first time to Israel, together with his companion, and fulfilled a long-term ambition to swim in the Dead Sea. And his choice of present? An iPad. It is exceptional to be so lively at 100, but if you reach 90 and are relatively free from the effects of disease, you will be able to live on your own, get about by public transport, maybe even still drive a car, and take a lively interest in current affairs. At the age of 90, the pianist Menahem Pressler played Mozart's piano concerto number 23 to rapturous applause in Oxford's Sheldonian Theatre and, for an encore, a Schubert *Moment Musical* – no score, just memory and perfect co-ordination.

So how is it that we all know 'old' 60-year-olds and sprightly 80-year-olds – people who seem 'old' beyond their years and others who we're convinced have a Dorian Gray style portrait in the attic? There is, of course, no denying that the ageing process exists and that there are only two phases in life:

- growing and developing

- ageing.

The turning point varies from person to person, but it can start in our teens, although for most of us it starts in the late twenties. The typical shape of the curve is shown overleaf.

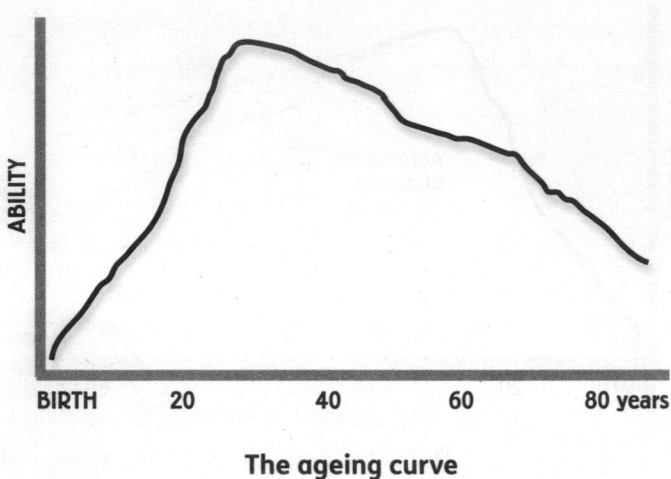

The ageing curve

Beware the fitness gap

The curve above shows the rate of loss of ability due to ageing alone. This is the best possible rate of decline. Unfortunately, the rate at which we lose strength to, for example, climb a steep slope, is likely to be quicker than this. In our thirties and forties, the point at which our physical attributes begin to diminish and the rate at which that actually proceeds are determined by loss of fitness. The difference between the best possible rate of decline and a person's actual rate of decline is what I call the *fitness gap* (see opposite).

I first described the fitness gap in an article in the *British Medical Journal* in 1982, when my work with older people in Oxford convinced me that, for many of them, their problems were caused or aggravated by inactivity and loss of fitness.

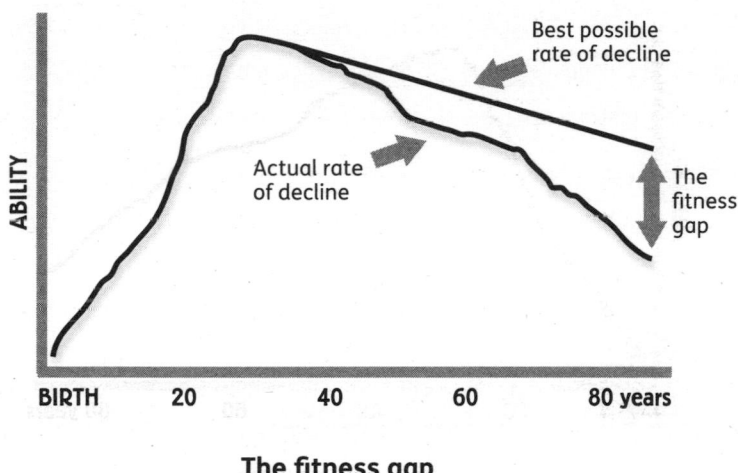

The fitness gap

The rate at which we lose fitness is determined by social factors, by the decisions we make about our life and the pressures that influence us.

People such as professional tennis players who commit themselves to fitness can often stay at the top until their early thirties, but it is around this age that our bodies begin to decline, even with full-time training. Think of stars like Roger Federer. Everything seemed to be going wrong for the seven-time winner at Wimbledon in 2013 when he was aged 32, but he turned his form around and reached the final again in 2014. Bradley Wiggins won the Tour de France in 2012 at the age of 31. Chris Froome won the Tour de France at the age of 27 in 2013, and the team coach said afterwards that 'it is impossible to say how many Tours Chris will win, he has all the physical and mental attributes for this race if nothing drastic changes for

5

quite some time'. Poor Froome had to drop out of the 2014 Tour de France as a consequence of a crash, so good luck is needed as well as good fitness.

Even for professional sports people the ageing process starts to kick in, for example, with a reduction in the maximal heart rate, essential for top athletes, of one per cent every year. For most people, however, decline starts earlier because they develop a less active lifestyle, for example, by buying a car, settling down and giving up football. Research published in 2014 showed that, for many men, fitness declined after marriage, principally because they put on weight. For many people who gave up sport and took up smoking in their teens, the decline starts much earlier.

Once our fitness decline has started, the rate is determined by social pressures. My first job in the public health service, for example, required me to own a car, whereas I had lived on my bike until then. With each job promotion, it's often the case that the amount of time spent in meetings and driving increases. Although this is definitely changing, there may well still be a feeling that it is not proper, in more senior positions, to turn up at work sweating, having cycled to the office.

There are two important points about the fitness gap. The first is that an inability to climb stairs at the age of 80, or get to the toilet in time, could be solely the result of loss of fitness, not the ageing process. When you are young, lack of fitness only affects your lifestyle

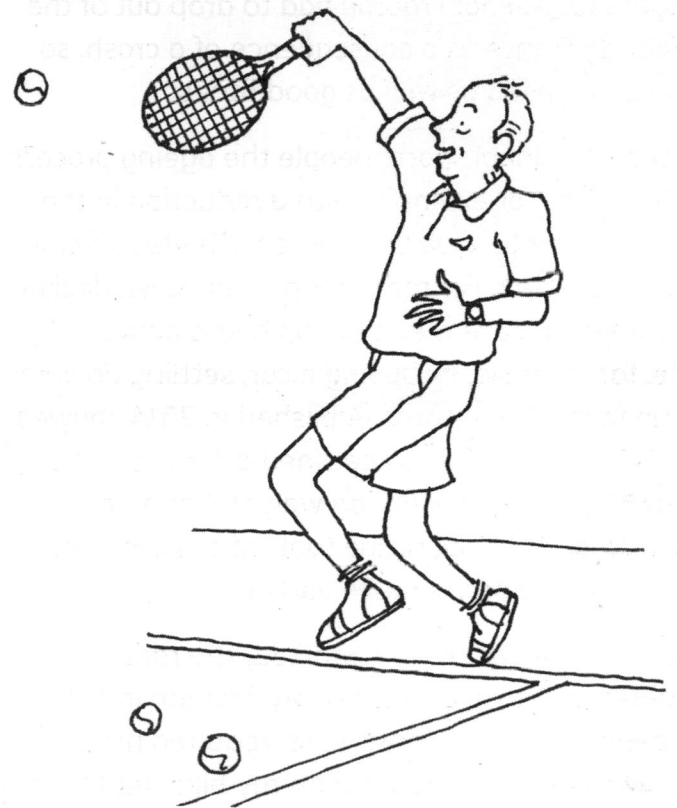

if you want to play tennis or football, but later on it can make the difference between dependence and independence.

The second important point, and the good news, is that the fitness gap can be narrowed *at any age*. And you're in luck – this book shows you how to go about narrowing the gap by improving your fitness. Chapter 2 tells you how to do it.

The other major factor that reduces our ability is disease.

Ageing and disease are different processes

Ageing is a complex process that is not yet fully understood. There is a genetic component, but, with a few exceptions, the risk of disease, and therefore how long we live, is determined more by lifestyle and environment than by genes.

If we study different age groups of the population, the percentage of people free from disease decreases as age increases. To put it another way, the number of new cases of disease increases with age. Furthermore, in each group from the age of 60 onwards, the percentage of people who have more than one disease increases.

This has led to the belief that ageing causes disease, but this is not the case. Most disease occurs as a result of living in an unhealthy environment or with an unhealthy lifestyle, and the longer you are exposed to it, the more likely it is that disease will develop.

Take my own situation. I am a little bit breathless, but that is not because of ageing; it is almost certainly the result of:

- growing up in Glasgow in the filthy fogs before the Clean Air Act of 1956

- having two parents who smoked Players cigarettes

- suffering a severe attack of measles before antibiotics were used to prevent complications

- suffering a small heart attack at the age of 67.

All in all I am lucky only to be a little breathless and still able to cycle three miles to the station. The only way to be certain of avoiding all the diseases that occur in older age groups – the only certain step – is not to reach old age!

In short, there are three important points about the relationship between disease and ageing:

- first, disease prevention is effective, not just for young people but for people in their fifties, sixties and seventies. Even at the age of 70 it is possible to postpone the onset of disease, or even prevent it occurring at all, by taking measures such as stopping smoking and losing weight

- second, you need a little bit of luck. Some people will develop disease even if they have no risk factors!

- third, your beliefs and attitudes about health and ageing play a very important part in both disease prevention and improving fitness.

Chapter 3 will show you ways to reduce your risk of disease, while chapter 4 will help you make decisions about healthcare that are right for you.

What you believe matters

In addition to the three pronged attack of ageing, disease and loss of fitness, there is a fourth element to all this – the social and psychological effects of growing old. For too many people, the social process is one in which we become slower, more cautious, less interested in the world around us, living more in the past and lamenting the passing of 'the good old days'. We all know someone like this, but they have probably always been more negative and pessimistic in their attitude. In addition, some of the changes that occur, and the depression that may come with them, are the result of being too influenced by the prevailing negative stereotype of old age.

But that doesn't have to be the case. Why should we be affected by an outmoded view of the older generation? It's time to take action! The facts of life are that our later years are not just a waiting game – decline is not inevitable! In fact, the older you get, the greater the need for a positive mental attitude and some positive action.

The seventies manifesto

This book is a call to arms. Become more active, mentally and physically; get more involved; help other people more and you will succeed in gaining better health. For many people this will need a change of attitude, and the meaning of the word attitude has changed in recent years. Our generation has always put an adjective before the word attitude. We say people have a positive attitude or an optimistic attitude, for example, but young people just use the word alone. They say a person has 'attitude', pronounced with a slight American accent, and 'attitude' in this sense means not only that they are positive but also that they know what they want and you don't want to mess with them. At 70 we all need a bit more attitude!

Finally you need a bit of luck. Menahem Pressler told me that the reason he was still able to play concertos on the international circuit was luck – not only luck with his genes (he still does not need glasses), but luck to have *music to give my life meaning*. We cannot all play an instrument to concert performance standard, but we can all find meaning in life – for example, by caring for grandchildren or other family members, or friends, or working either for extra income or as a volunteer. For Pressler, the best thing, his luck, comes not from playing to packed concert halls but from teaching. You can make your own luck and chapter 5 will emphasise the importance of finding meaning.

So make today the day you decide to make some changes – have a look through some of the recommendations in this book – even if you don't manage to adopt all of them. Even small changes can make a big difference to your fitness, outlook and attitude to the next chapter in your life!

2

DON'T WORRY – GET FITTER!

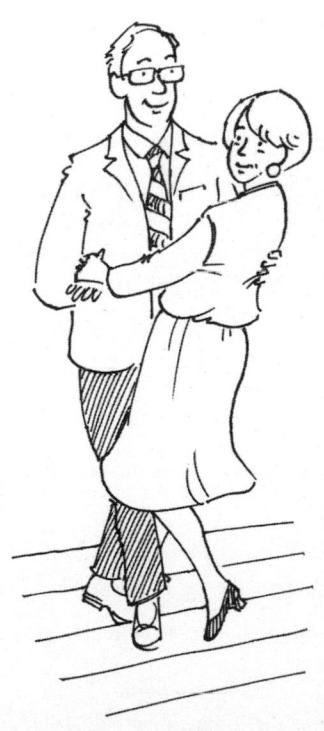

Use it or lose it!

Fitness ... what pictures does this word conjure up? Lycra, the gym, weights, sweat? These are the images that alarm many of us, but fitness is not something just for 'young' people; as we saw in the last chapter, fitness is far more important for people in their seventies than for people in their twenties. The young only need to think about fitness if they want to take part in sport, but *everyone* who is 70 needs to focus on fitness.

As we saw in chapter 1:

- there are only two phases of life: the phase of growth and development, and the phase of ageing

- for most of us, the age at which the phase of ageing begins is determined by social factors which change our behaviour, not biological ageing

- the ability to do things at any age is not only affected by the effects of ageing but also by our level of fitness – that is, by the size of our fitness gap.

Many of us aged 70 or 75 can probably do everything we want to do – go upstairs, for example, or bend to tie shoelaces. However, we all need to think ahead.

For people in their eighties, fitness becomes of vital importance because it can make the difference between being able to dress unaided or not, or being able to reach the toilet in time when nature calls urgently. The importance of this has never been appreciated by the medical profession.

In the 1980s I was part of a study looking at medical students' knowledge of the benefits of exercise in older age, compared with their knowledge about diet. Their lack of knowledge was lamentable, and we published our recommendations in a chapter called 'The Risks of Inactivity' in my book *Prevention of Disease in the Elderly*. We covered the whole age range from 60 upwards, but it was clear that most of the serious problems, particularly those that result in dependence on others occur in your eighties and nineties. Many of them are the consequence of disease combined with the progressive loss of fitness that has occurred since the age of 20 and health can deteriorate even more quickly when someone becomes inactive. These problems usually result in referral to the NHS or social services.

We have not repeated our study of medical students but I don't think we would find much difference even today. It is true that doctors and other health professionals are more active now than they were thirty years ago and appreciate the benefits of exercise and fitness for themselves, but many are still keener to prescribe drugs alone rather than recommend a new exercise regime to work alongside them.

Of course, there are a few exceptions. Cardiologists now ensure that you get advice on exercise the day after you have had a heart attack. Geriatricians – specialists in older patients – know that although it is more difficult to regain 'lost' abilities, such as recovering your balance if you stumble and walking quickly enough to get to the toilet in time, in your eighties, it is still possible. You can even do it in your nineties (and beyond).

The specialty of geriatrics emerged about fifty years ago when a group of doctors decided that it was wrong to write off elderly people who had more than one condition in the way that other specialists did. They believed not only in caring for older people but also in helping them regain their abilities. This was a new philosophy. Today most of their work is with people in their eighties and nineties but their influence on medicine has been great. These days it is GPs who provide most support to people in their seventies, and they and their nursing colleagues now provide not only diagnosis and treatment but also encouragement to believe in your potential to get healthier and stay healthy.

And there's research to back this up. A project in 2014 found that people with a sedentary lifestyle and reduced mobility showed a significant improvement in mobility and independence by participating in a home exercise programme. If you take action to get fitter every year during your fifties, sixties and seventies, you will reach the age of 80 or 90 in a much better physical and mental condition. There is no guarantee that fitness training will extend your life, but for most of us the aim is not a longer life, whatever the quality, but a shorter period of disability and dependency at the end, with a good death to complete a good life.

Even if you develop some long-term condition like heart disease or cancer, fitness remains important – in fact, it becomes even more important. Because the onset of disease may reduce your ability to remain as active, you may lose fitness more quickly as a result. Heart disease is the only long-term condition in which exercise, particularly vigorous exercise, carries a risk. If you have heart disease, you and your doctor will have to balance the risks of exercise with the risks of inactivity. Back in the 'old days' it was common to recommend rest, but these days activity is increasingly promoted, and indeed prescribed. In most hospitals now, patients who have had a heart attack will have a consultation with

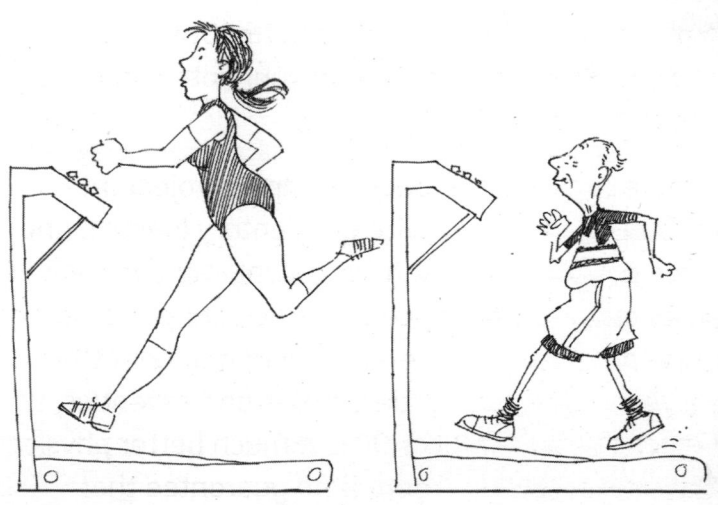

an exercise therapist before being discharged from hospital, and will be expected to turn up to a gym two weeks later to start their rehabilitation on the treadmill.

Other conditions cause different problems. For example, if you have had a stroke or developed severe arthritis, it makes movement more difficult. Physiotherapists are skilled in helping people with disabilities and can design an exercise programme that will help them recover strength, stamina, suppleness and skill, not just while they are attending the physiotherapy department but for the rest of their lives. Exercise is a powerful therapy.

What is fitness?

You can get some idea of fitness while you sit and read this by taking your pulse. The lower the pulse, the fitter you are – usually. However, on its own this is not a very good measure as some illnesses and prescribed drugs can result in a slow heart rate. For that reason, fitness is best measured by the degree to which the body is 'upset' when it is asked to do extra work, such as running upstairs or climbing a hill. Your fitness is revealed when you have to do something out of the ordinary. The fitter you are, the better you feel, and the less your body will have to change to cope with physical and psychological challenges.

But don't worry – whether you're a weekend hill climber, or the idea of a walk to the shops fills you with dread, the good news is that fitness can be improved at any age, and therefore the fitness gap can be reduced.

Getting fitter now, in your seventies, is the key – laying the foundations for when it becomes of vital importance to you in your eighties and nineties.

The 5S fitness programme

It might seem obvious, but I think it is important to reiterate that taking regular exercise in your seventies will make you feel better in your eighties. Fitness has five aspects, each associated with an 'S word':

- **s**tamina

- **s**trength

- **s**kill (balance)

- **s**uppleness

- p**s**ychology.

I can give advice but *you* have to take action. The time commitment from you is:

- a very doable ten minutes a day focused principally on strength, suppleness and skill

- three longer sessions every week, walking, cycling or dancing, focused primarily on stamina

- a daily mental workout.

The great thing about this investment of time is not only the long term benefit but the immediate one. Exercise helps you feel better immediately *and* the risks of increasing exercise are very small.

Is it safe to exercise?

There is no single medical condition which will be made worse by exercise of moderate intensity – even heart disease, which only fifty years ago was treated by 'rest' (partly because there were no effective treatments available). In fact, specialists are playing a leading part in promoting exercise as part of a recovery programme. So too are cancer specialists and their two big charities, the British Heart Foundation and Macmillan, are leading the campaign to build exercise into best medical practice and self care. Ask your GP, or speak to your pharmacist about it next time you go to collect your prescription.

INCREASING YOUR STAMINA

Stamina is primarily the result of the way your heart, lungs and muscles work together when walking, cycling – or mowing the grass! Having good stamina means you can also meet demands for extra oxygen when, for example, you have to climb stairs.

The easiest way to improve and maintain stamina is to increase the amount you walk and try to find ways of making yourself a little breathless each day, for example, by choosing the stairs instead of the lift. A

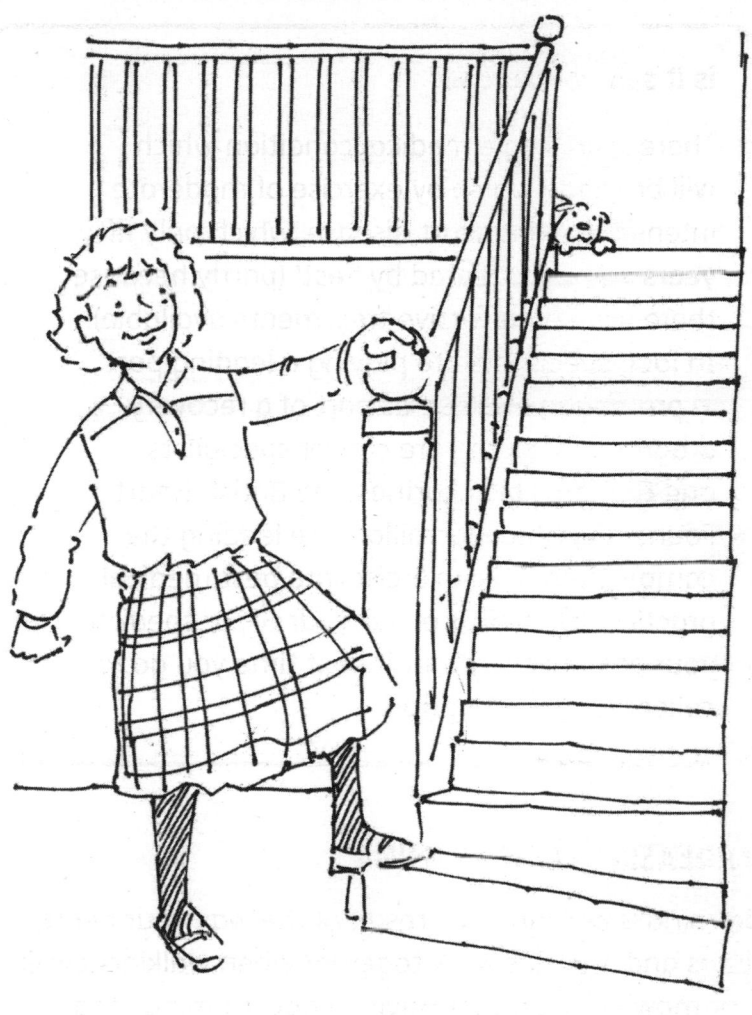

new campaign called Step Jockey is posting reminder notices beside lifts; so use the stairs whenever possible, at least to go up (many people find lifts good for going down if they have knee problems!). Make a resolution such as the one overleaf:

21

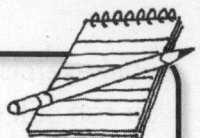

From now on I will:

- walk or cycle for long enough to get a little breathless, on at least three days a week

- go swimming or dancing, or play tennis, bowls or golf, or do something that makes me breathless at least once a week.

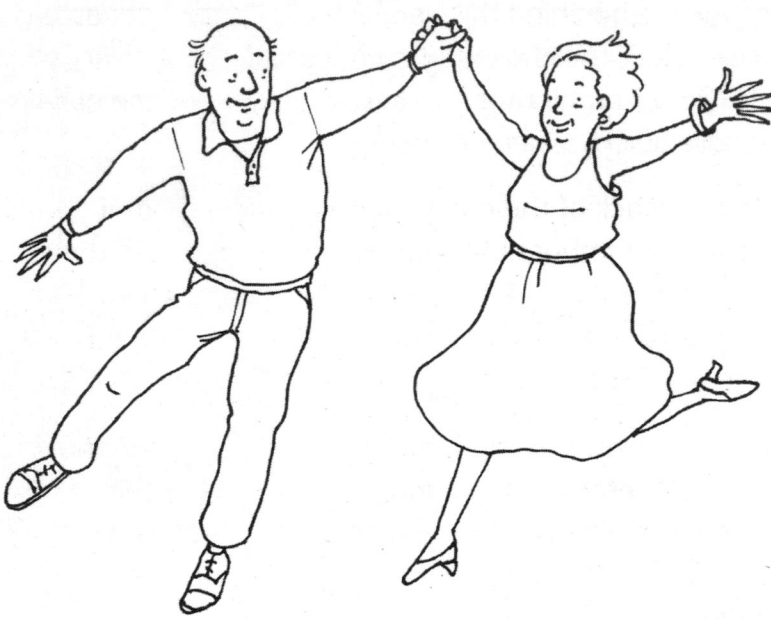

Traditionally people have recommended thirty minutes as the required time for walking, and, if you can do it, thirty minutes walking is a good duration, every day if you can manage it but on at least three days a week. Lack of time, however, should not be an excuse to avoid exercise because even if you are working flat out you can still redesign your day to fit in more walking, by parking further away from your work for example. Of course, some health problems do limit the length of time you can walk. Fortunately, there is increasing research interest in the greater benefits that can result from shorter, more intense exercise, captured in a *Daily Express* headline in July 2014:

TWO MINUTES EXERCISE A WEEK CAN BEAT AGEING

The research behind this headline points out that as we get older the challenge is not so much the ability to walk for thirty minutes at a leisurely pace but the ability to *move quickly when necessary.*

The drawback of the thirty minute target is that it might seem impossibly daunting for someone in their nineties, but it is better to do some exercise, even ten minutes at moderate intensity, at any age than it is not to do any exercise at all.

But what exactly is moderate intensity exercise? This has to be determined by you, by the effect of the exercise on you. The best indicator is your breathing. Ambling along, admiring the view, stopping as soon as you feel a tiny bit breathless, is a perfectly acceptable way of passing the time but it won't improve your physical fitness. You need to feel a change in your breathing, not so much that you can't talk but certainly enough to know you are working a little, or, to put it another way, it is doing you good. If you notice your breathing increasing, your heart rate will also increase. And don't worry – you don't need to measure your pulse as you walk (which can attract well meaning but annoying enquiries from passers by!)

For years the message has been to do thirty minutes of walking or cycling or swimming to improve stamina, but it is now clear that people in their seventies can really benefit even from ten minutes of physical activity. The trick here is to *build exercise into everyday life* so that it doesn't feel like a 'chore' – and little things make a big difference – for example, by taking stairs two steps at a time or by getting off the bus one or two stops early.

So that's a look at stamina; remember the mantra – get up and out to get your breathing rate up and your heart pumping faster *three days a week*. It's what you choose to do that makes it enjoyable. Hitting the gym and grinding out minutes on the treadmill can be dull – yes, I absolutely agree – but use your imagination! Take the dog for a walk (or borrow a friend's). Take up a new sport – if you've always fancied learning tennis, now's the time! If you already play tennis, ask for lessons as a present and try to play better, faster. Whether it's cycling to the station, going for a swim, walking briskly to the shops and carrying the shopping back, or meeting a friend to go dancing or bowling, remember, it's not a punishment. Being active, getting outdoors, going to meet friends and playing sports – all of this is fun!

These boots were made for walking

Walking is such a good, easy, safe and inexpensive way of preventing loss of fitness and getting fitter. Here are my top tips to walk your way fitter.

We're fighting a Sitting Down Epidemic. We eat more and richer food. And we're using our bodies less – we drive, sit at work, sit when out meeting friends, sit to watch TV. Along with the other ideas mentioned so far, fight back and take action with the simplest form of defence: walking.

Walking is wonderful, the best exercise there is, and it's free! It gets you out in the elements and really gets your body moving. Walk in the park, to the shops, the post office, the bank. Walk with a friend, walk on your own and use the time to phone people or catch up with messages, or to listen to the radio on your mobile – use it for 'you time'. Whatever you use it for, remember that the benefits are mostly for the lower limbs and for improving stamina, the aspect of fitness that allows you to exercise or do gardening or run for a bus without getting breathless. Don't forget the other elements of our exercise programme – of which more next – which will build up your upper body strength, balance and suppleness too!

As I've said, even a brisk ten minute walk is good for you but, if you can manage, walk for thirty minutes a day.

- if you are too busy, for example, driving to look after grandchildren (themselves of course a useful antidote to sitting), you may have to divide that thirty minutes into two blocks. For example, park your car fifteen minutes away from where you have to go, not as close as possible.

- use public transport instead of your car wherever possible. The walk to the bus stop is part of your quota!

- if you can only walk for ten minutes at a time, that's fine too – try to walk for ten minutes three times a day. Once you keep a tally you easily start thinking this way – for example, taking a ten minute walk after breakfast and then ten minutes after lunch and ten minutes in the evening; routinely, obsessively, every day.

And think about what you're wearing on your feet – comfy shoes are a must, but you can also get shoes that look good and are good for walking so you don't need to wear clumpy boots (unless in the mud or on a mountain).

Walk tall

We all know how to walk, but don't forget your posture. We all need to reduce the forward stoop that is so common and so often portrayed as the image of older people on those infuriating 'old stooped people crossing' road traffic signs for example. It is easy to slip into this posture when walking, letting your head and shoulders drop forward like a tortoise. What you need to do is to be conscious of your posture. Don't stick your chin out like a caricature of a guardsman. Imagine instead that there is a line attached to the crown of your skull and drawn vertically upwards. Then just draw your shoulders back and you have good posture. I often ask regular walking companions to say 'posture, posture, posture' and poke me in the side if they see me slipping into tortoise mode.

Walking with a stick, or two

A stick is often seen as a sign of decrepitude but it needn't be – hikers have always carried a trusty stave and this is coming back into fashion. Nordic walking is the name given to walking with a good pole, the Nordic walking pole is a modified skiing pole with a rubber tip. Ask for one, or two, for your birthday and use them with pride. They reduce the risk of falling, increase the number of calories you burn up, improve your posture and are handy for dealing with aggressive dogs!

Thought for the day

For at least part of your regular walk, say ten minutes, fix your eyes on a particular point and concentrate on that point, on your posture and on your breathing. Empty your mind of other thoughts and worries, and just *be*. Measure it with respect to a couple of landmarks, two trees for example, so that you recognise when it's time to have this period of mindful meditation. Try to do this along the same route every day so that it becomes part of your mental health programme (see pages 63 and 175).

Into the great outdoors

Whenever you can, regularly if possible, get close to nature when you walk – it may not always be possible, but a turn around your local park is a great way to bring a little tranquillity to your day.

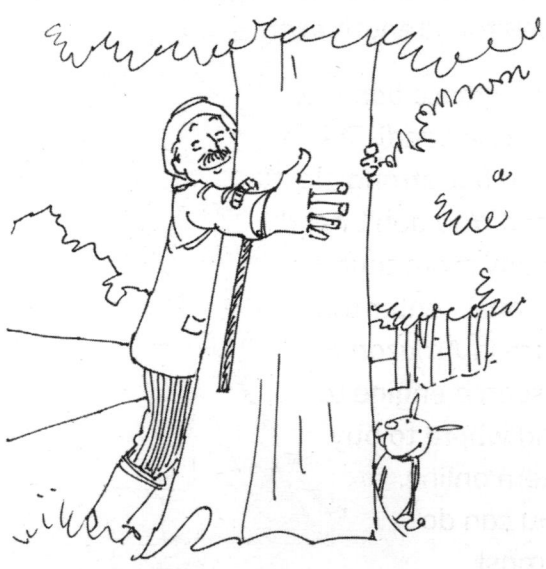

We're working up a sweat, but it's also important to spend at least ten minutes a day on the three other 's's I mentioned earlier – strength, skill and suppleness.

INCREASING YOUR STRENGTH

With a bit of luck, a clever friend will have given you some fitness equipment for your seventieth birthday, but, if not, you should consider buying two items to increase and maintain muscle strength:

- *a pair of dumbbells,* 1kg, 3kg or 5kg – or all three! You should not need to pay more than £12 for each pair. Weights are best for strengthening your upper limbs, forearms, arms and shoulders. We're not talking about bulking up here – you won't get an Arnold Schwarzenegger body overnight – and these exercises are just as important for women as for men (see pages 38–9 for strength exercises).

- *a resistance band (or exercise band).* This is like a big, strong elastic band. You don't need to pay more than £3 for one – enter the term in Amazon or a search engine to find where to buy them online. You can do almost everything with a fitness band that you can do with weights, and they are much easier to pack! There are lots of exercises on the web and you can make up your own. See page 40–1 for ideas.

BALANCING SKILLS

I think the most important skill to maintain and improve is the *ability to keep upright*. Falls increase in frequency after the age of 70, and most of them occur in the home.

So why are we more likely to fall as we get older? There are four main culprits:

- our sense of balance gets worse as we age, partly because of a deterioration of our inner ear, sometimes as a side effect of medication (e.g. blood pressure medication)

- muscles get weaker and can't quickly recover the vertical position

- we lose our ability to co-ordinate all the actions that need to work together to steady ourselves when we trip or stumble

- poor lighting, loose floor coverings and other hazards in the home.

All types of sport and active hobbies are helpful in the fight to stay upright. You might go dancing, for example, or sign up for a local environmental improvement scheme. Activity helps the brain co-ordinate muscles,

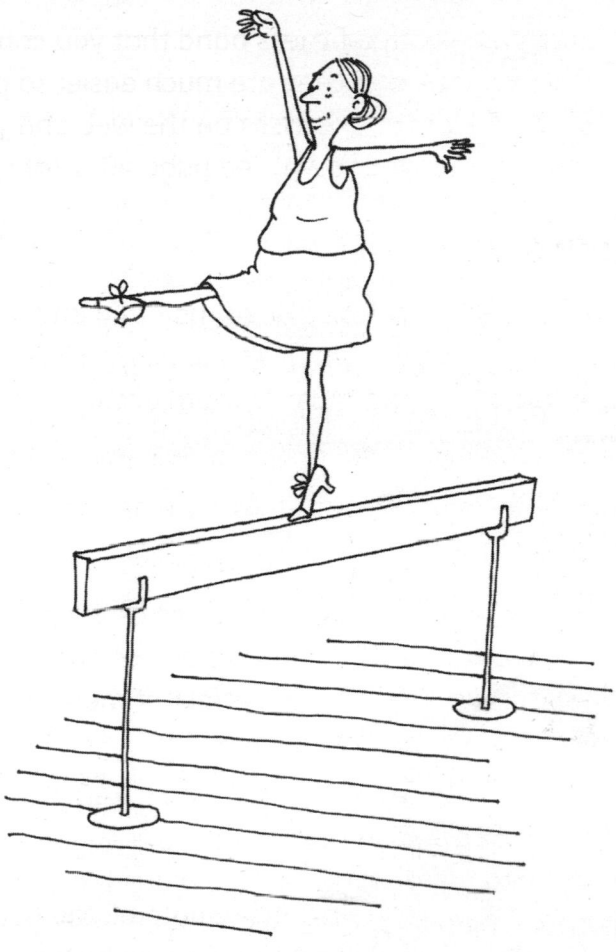

which in turn improves movement. But there are specific ways you can improve your balance, and your ability to recover from a stumble, and so reduce your risk of falls and fractures.

There are two pieces of action you can take – the first is to reduce your risk of falling (see page 47), and the second is to reduce your rate of bone loss (see page 98).

31

INCREASING YOUR SUPPLENESS

If you look at a chicken leg or, even better, a leg of lamb, you will see a white, shiny tissue that divides the red bundles of muscle fibres and connects them to the bones just near the joints. This white tissue is a mixture of elastin and collagen. It does lose some elasticity as a result of ageing, as the balance of elastin to collagen decreases, but the good news is that most of the loss of suppleness is due to loss of fitness through inactivity, not to ageing – so we can all do something about it.

Suppleness is probably the most under-valued part of fitness and the bit that is most important as we age. Much of the sport and training we do as younger people focuses on strength, stamina and skill, not on suppleness, and it shows. To regain and increase suppleness you need to stretch your joints and muscles.

Here is a simple exercise to increase your shoulder suppleness. Standing erect, with good posture, put your right hand round on your left shoulder cupping the shoulder; now just push the hand a bit further on to the left shoulder blade, push and relax, push and relax. Then repeat on the other side.

Here is another – hold on to the back of the sofa, or grab the kitchen counter, or the rail along the landing if you have one. Stand with your knees shoulder width apart, now sink down, bending your hips and knees until you can feel a sense of stretching. Hold it there for

a count of ten, then come back up an inch or two.
Go down and up ten times, slowly.

Planning your Daily Ten Minutes Triple S Programme (Strength, Suppleness and Skill)

CHOOSE YOUR TIMING

It doesn't matter when you exercise and it doesn't
matter what you wear, as long as it's comfortable –
it's often easiest to exercise in pyjamas or a nightie.
It therefore might be simplest to do it first thing in the
morning, but not everyone feels up to it first thing.
Find the right time of day for *you*. The key is to focus
on ten minutes a day and I find it helps to stick to the
same time of day, every day – because it becomes
second nature. If you prefer, you can do your weekly
allocation of seventy minutes in five episodes of
fourteen minutes, or six of twelve, but it is better to do
ten minutes every day and not to think about having 'a
day off'. Remember what Olympic gold medallist Daley
Thompson said when he was asked if he took Christmas
Day off: 'Of course not, I train twice on Christmas Day
because I know others aren't training at all!' Besides,
you will want to try out your new exercise bands or
weights that your friends and family have given you
for Christmas!

Exercise is not a punishment. It should be a joy because
it will make each day better, so stick to the daily
programme! It is good to be obsessed about doing the

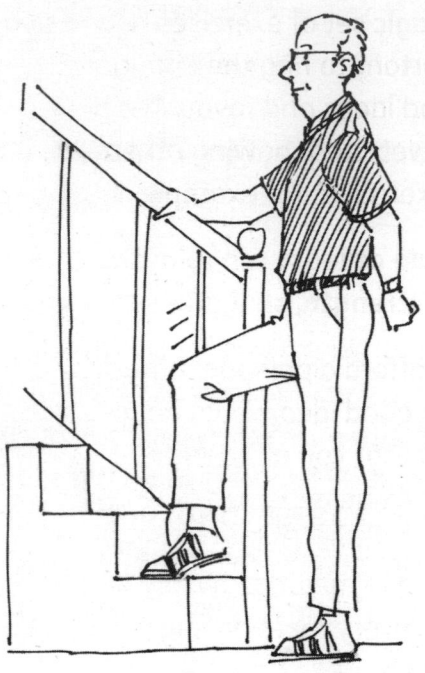

ten minutes, and even aim to increase the time you spend on it very slightly as you get older:

- when you reach 71 the programme becomes the 71-minute programme – on one day you will do an extra minute of training.

- when you are 72 you will be on the 72-minute programme – on two days you will do eleven minutes. And so on until...

- when you are 80, you will be doing eleven minutes a day on four days of the week, and twelve minutes on three days a week – work it out!

There is no magic set of exercises and to avoid boredom it is very important to ring the changes. I've given you some good ideas and favourites here, but there are excellent websites showing others – just type 'suppleness exercises', for example, into a search engine.

The key is to do at least ten minutes of these exercises for strength, skill and suppleness every day.

If you cannot afford a personal fitness instructor or Pilates tutor, a good idea would be to suggest to your club or society that you all contribute towards a special meeting with a fitness instructor to show you exercises and answer questions. Or it might be that you can reinforce the triple message by building warm-ups and stretching into every meeting, even if its primary function is bridge or bowls.

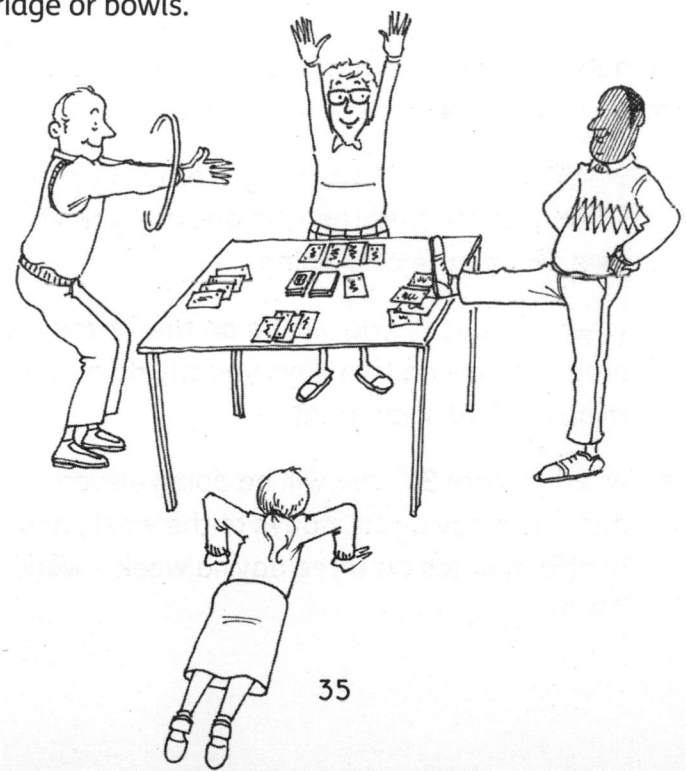

35

So what are we trying to improve with the Daily Ten Minute Triple S programme?

1. shoulder flexibility – not just the joints but also shoulder blades and chest muscles

2. flexibility of our neck – forward, back and side-to-side

3. strength of our upper limbs – the lower limbs are often kept strong by walking and cycling, but most of us need to work on upper limb strength

4. spinal strength, stability and flexibility of our 'core' muscles (see page 42 for more on core stability)

5. flexibility of our hips – again, forward, back and side to side

6. flexibility of the knees

7. stretchability of the muscles at the back of the lower limbs (the hamstrings above the knee, the calf muscles below)

8. better balance.

None of these exercises need any equipment, except to increase the strength of your arms (see page 38). At least four of your ten minutes of exercise should focus on suppleness.

FOR SUPPLE SHOULDERS

Circle your arms backwards, trying
to brush your ears as the arms pass.
If you have frozen shoulder, you
might not be able to do this at first,
but try it gently. Don't cause yourself
pain; you will probablyfind this
a deceptively simple but challenging
exercise at first.

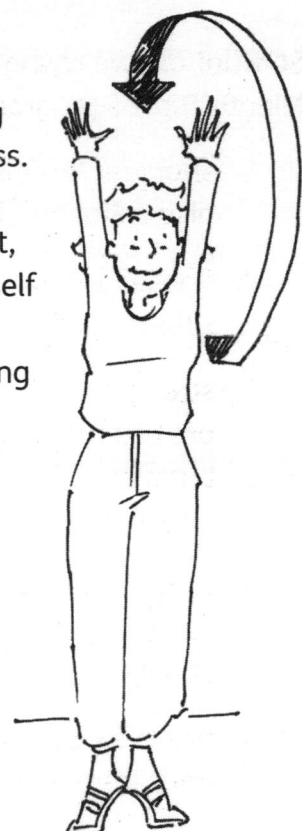

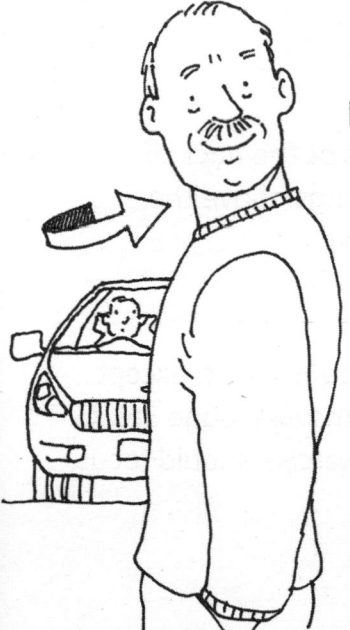

FOR A SUPPLE NECK

Circle your head on your neck
slowly; don't push it with your
hands. Look right and left over
each shoulder as though you
were checking for an overtaking
car. Don't forget your posture:
imagine a wire from the crown
of your head to the ceiling. Stand
straight, chin in, not like a tortoise
with its head forward and chin out.

37

FOR UPPER LIMB STRENGTH

Dumbbells, or weights, are the right tools for both forearms and biceps. Exercise bands are also good, and so too is the humble press-up! Create your own variations if you are finding they get boring after a while, but here are three starters:

- stand up straight, good posture, hands by your side, weight in each hand

- lift your arms out to your sides slowly until horizontal and slowly lower them again, don't lose control

- do this ten times, rest then repeat.

The trick is to keep the weights beside the remote control for the television so that every time you reach for the remote to look at the weather forecast you do this exercise while still watching it.

- with a 1kg or 3kg weight in your right hand stand upright, let your hand hang beside your body

- bend your elbow until your forearm is upright, now let your hand drop down slowly, always in control

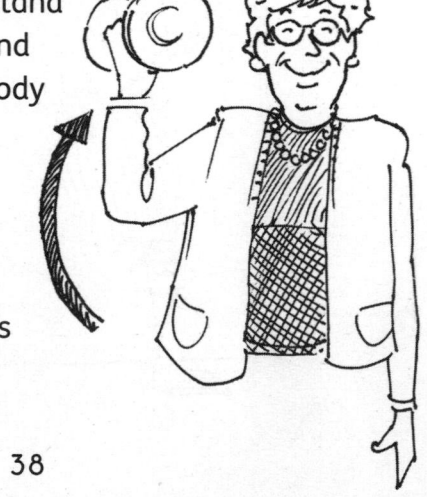

- change to the left hand and repeat

- now take the same weight in your right hand at shoulder height

- push up gently until your arm is straight

- count to ten then lower it again, slowly

- repeat five times, then give the left arm the same treatment.

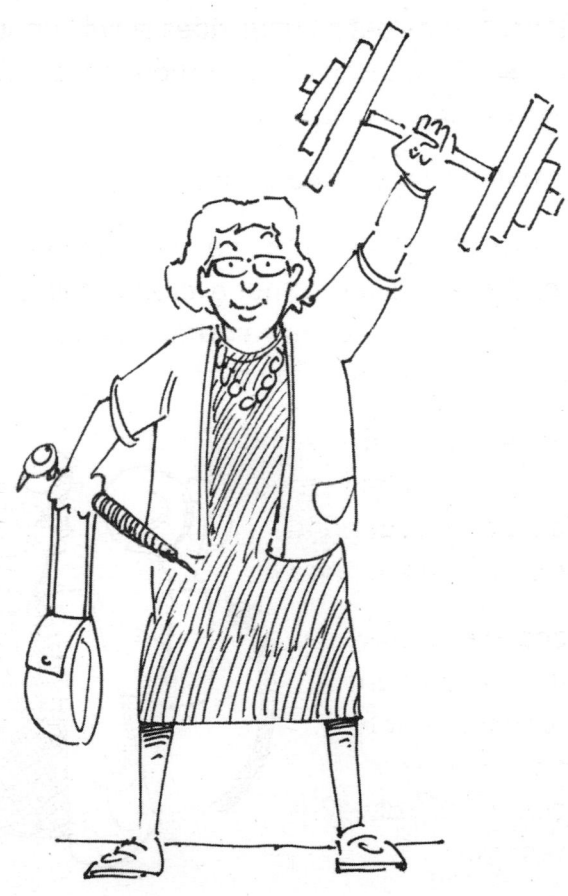

The fitness band is wonderful for upper body strength. Here are a couple of ideas:

- using your right hand, hold the band vertically down your back

- now put your left hand behind your back, forearm horizontal, as though a policeman had your arm behind your back and grasp the band at waist level

- Put a little tension on the band and, when you are ready stretch your right arm above your head. Keep the band as straight as you can for a few seconds. Then, slowly, lower it again. Repeat.

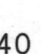

- Change arms and repeat the exercise

- to make it harder, shorten the length of the band between your two hands.

Use the band like an old-fashioned chest expander:

- Stand up straight, good posture and grip the band with both hands, arms straight out in front of you

- now pull your arms apart until the band is flat across your chest, hold it for a few seconds, then move slowly back to the original position.

This is very good for chest and shoulder muscles. Remember you will need to find the level of resistance that is right for you and that is determined by how far apart your hands are when you grip the band – the closer together they are the harder it is to stretch the band.

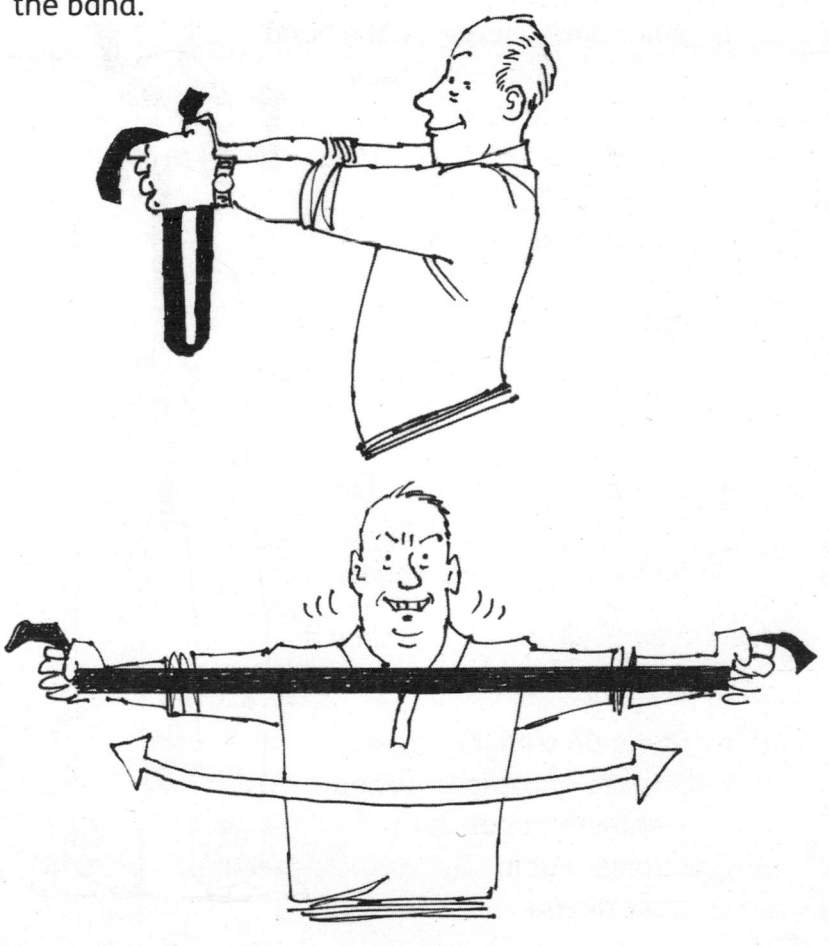

FOR CORE BODY STRENGTH

Lie on your back, hands behind your head, and then bend forward lifting your head and shoulders up six inches and hold that position, count to twenty if you can, and aim to build up to twenty seconds over a month if you can't.

Secondly, with hands by your sides, lift your feet six inches off the ground, keeping your legs straight: hold them up for twenty seconds if you can, or build up to that over a month if you can't. Then, criss-cross your legs ten times, before lowering them slowly. These exercises are good for abdominal muscles, they help with posture and prevent back ache. They also reduce the risk of a hernia developing in the groin. If you already have a hernia, ask your doctor which is the best exercise for you.

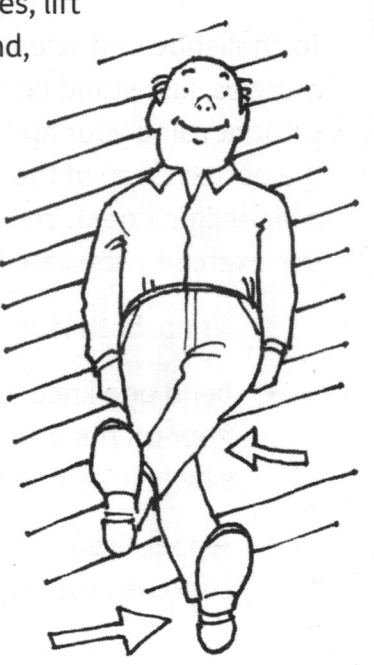

FOR YOUR HIPS

Lie on your back with your right knee bent and your right foot on the floor. Rest your left ankle across the knee of the bent leg. Push gently on the left knee and rock the knee a little away from you, keeping the left knee pointing towards the wall. Do this ten times, then repeat the exercise with the other leg.

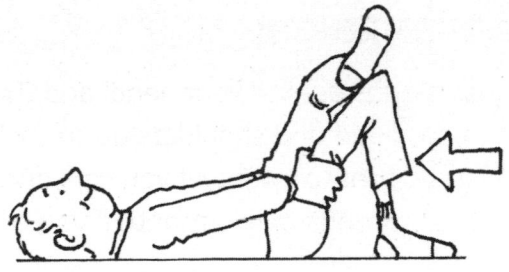

To challenge and strengthen your hips and thigh muscles, just stand up from sitting on a chair ten times without using your arms; if this is too easy, do it from the bottom step of the stairs instead. (If you have had a hip replacement, check with your doctor before doing this exercise.) You could also try this simple exercise:

- sit up, both legs straight out in front of you

- bend one knee, now try to put that foot on the floor on the other side of the straight leg. Count slowly to ten.

- repeat five times, then change legs, This stretches the tissues round your hip joints.

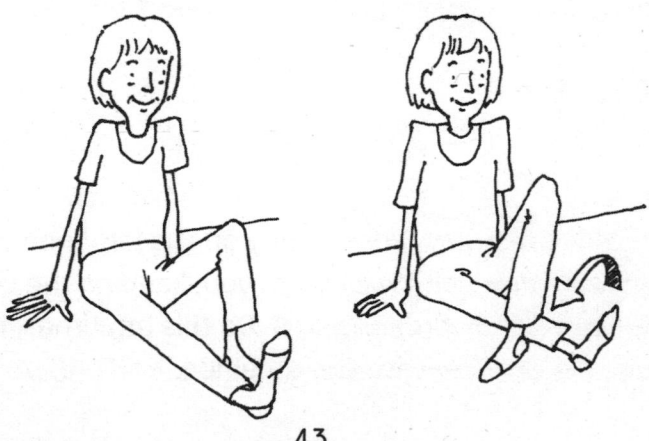

43

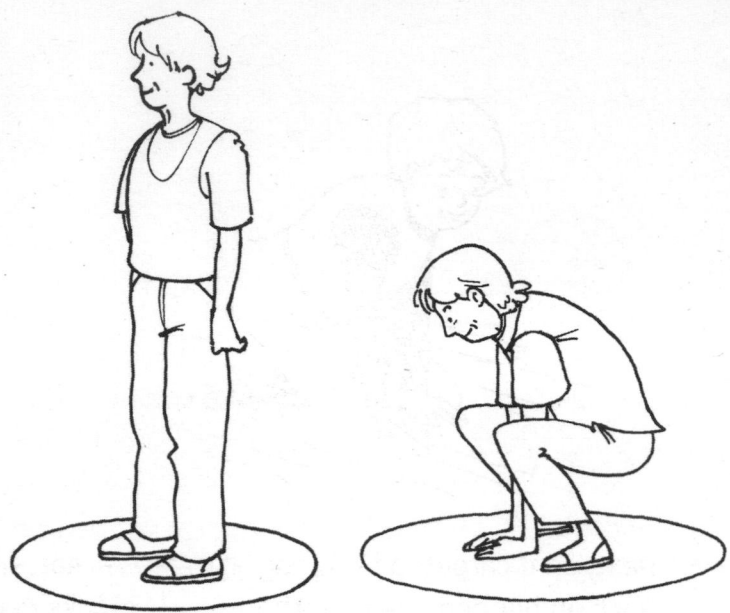

FOR YOUR KNEES

- first, stand with feet shoulder width apart. Then bend your knees and hips and try to touch the floor with your fingertips without bending your back too much. A little arching is unavoidable.

- if you can do this, try to put your palms on the floor

- do this ten times, then put your feet three inches further apart and do another ten, and then go for another ten.

Doing this ten times quite quickly is good for both hips and knees, stretching both muscles and ligaments. This should not cause discomfort. If putting your palms on the floor causes discomfort, go back to the fingertips.

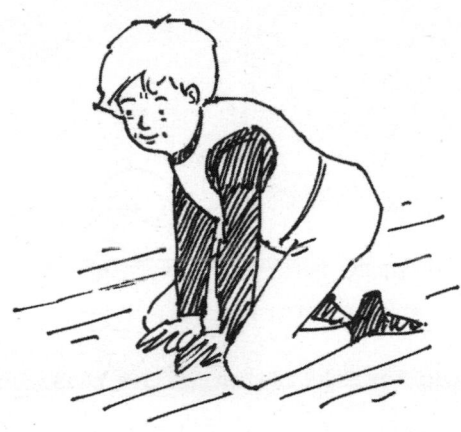

- next, on a carpeted floor, rug or exercise mat, sit back on bended knees so that your buttocks rest on your heels, if you can

- if you can't get your buttocks to rest on your heels get as near as you can and hold this position; it might help if you rest your hands on the floor in front of you.

You can build this into other daily routines, such as making the fire or clearing out a cupboard or listening to *The Archers*. (I find the key is never to listen to *The Archers* sitting down!) This increases the suppleness of the tendons and ligaments round the knee joints.

FOR STRETCHABLE HAMSTRINGS AND CALVES

- keeping your back straight, bend forward until you feel your hamstrings – the muscles at the back of the leg – really stretching

45

- hold while you count to ten, relax and stand up

- repeat this five times.

You can adapt this exercise to try and touch your toes, but this involves curving your back and should *not* be attempted by anyone with back problems.

- for stretchable calf muscles, stand arm's length from a low wall or a kitchen counter

- place both hands on top of the wall or counter

- put one foot back ten or twelve inches then put your back heel on the ground and feel the calf muscles of the back leg stretch. Count to ten. Repeat three times and then repeat with the other leg.

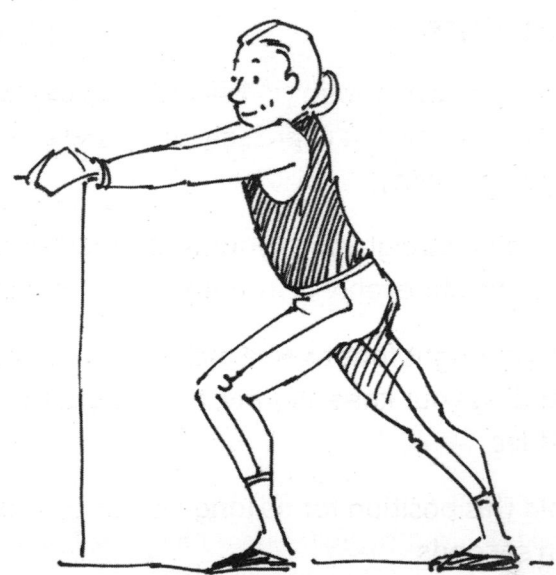

FOR STRONG FEET AND LEGS

The little muscles of the foot are supported by the tendons of the calf muscles, so you can do these two exercises to support your feet:

- firstly, put the front half of your right foot on a step

- hold on to something with one hand and bounce up and down very gently ten times

- repeat with the other foot.

Secondly, stand on your tiptoes for three minutes (I always watch or listen to the weather forecast on my toes). You might find it helpful to hold on to a chair or the edge of a basin or work surface while you do this.

BETTER BALANCE

You need to be both strong and skilful to avoid falling. Here is a simple balance exercise you should practise to improve your stability:

- stand up straight with your feet together and your weight evenly distributed on both feet

- lift your right foot twelve inches off the floor, bending your knee slightly, and balance on your left leg

- hold this position for as long as you can, aim for ten seconds

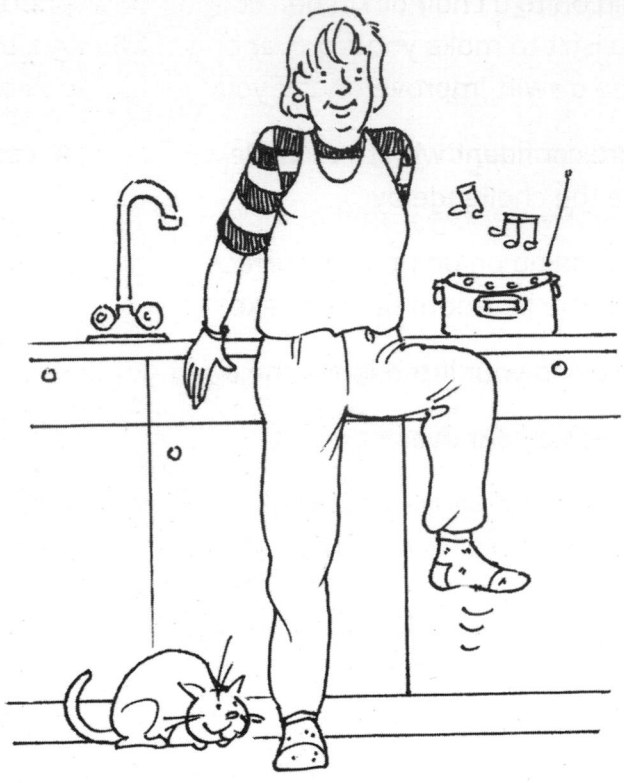

- repeat with your left leg

- if you can, repeat three times

- do this every day, and increase the time you hold your legs up every week.

As you do this exercise, focus on a spot straight ahead. Try to maintain good posture throughout by keeping your chest lifted, your shoulders down and back, and your abdominal muscles braced. Then breathe comfortably. If you feel a bit wobbly when you first try this, hold on to a chair or kitchen counter for support – the idea isn't to make you fall over on your first go, but you'll see a swift improvement if you practise each day.

If you are confident with this simple exercise, you can increase the challenge by:

- standing on an uneven surface (a crumpled towel on the bedroom floor, for example)

- waving your lifted leg in the air

- closing your eyes.

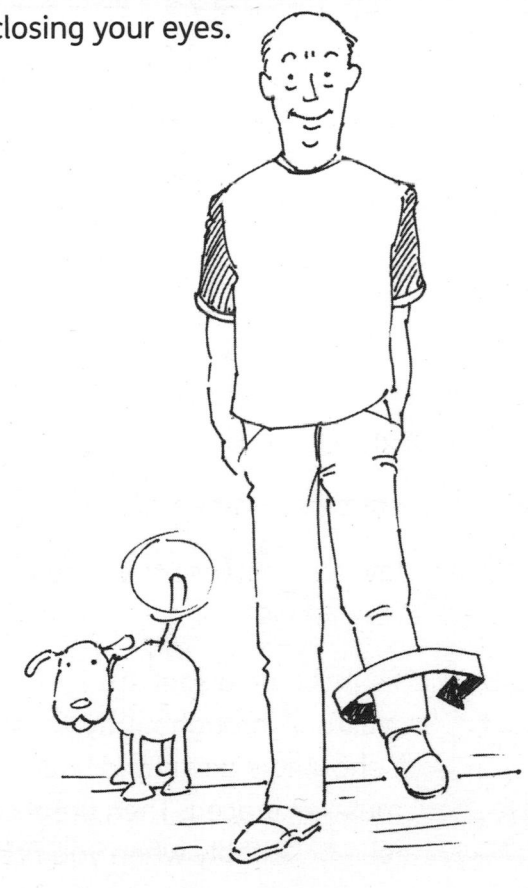

Just like the stamina section, the key is to make these simple exercises part of your day-to-day life. So, why not try standing on one leg when brushing your gums and teeth? Remember to have something you can hold on to if you feel unsteady, particularly if you close your eyes.

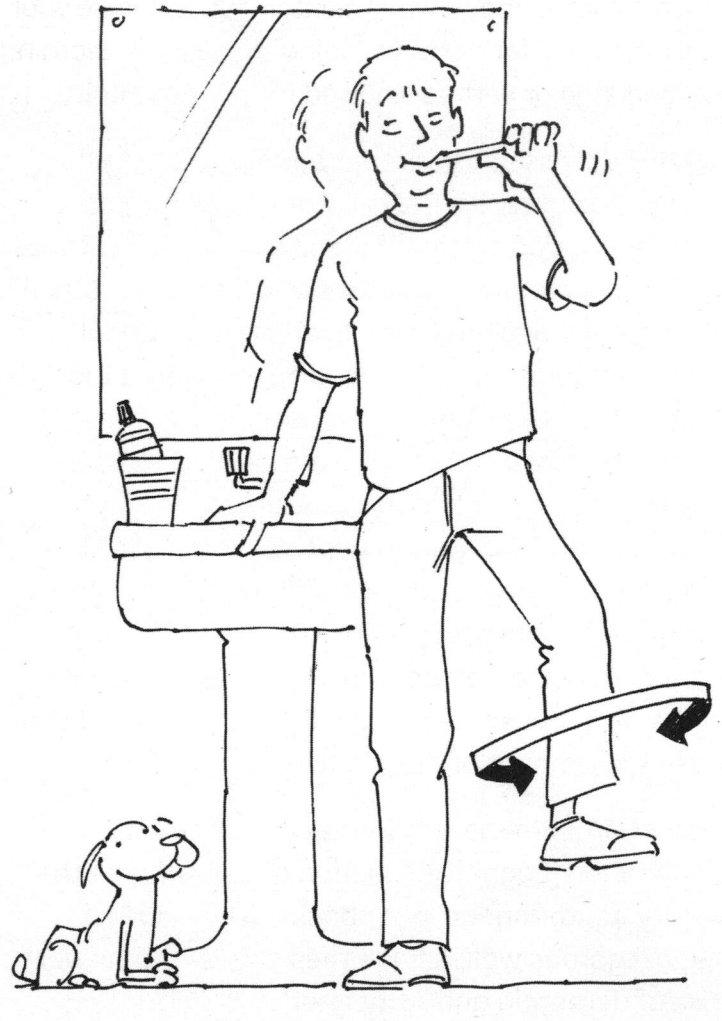

IMPROVE YOUR PSYCHOLOGICAL FITNESS

Mens sana in corpora sano – 'a healthy mind in a healthy body'. This old Latin proverb can be adapted for the twenty-first century to 'a fitter mind in a fitter body'. In the next chapter we will look more at the effects of ageing on the brain and some of its psychological or mental functions, and how to maintain and improve your mental fitness by, for example, doing crosswords, learning a new language or getting involved in the community.

But all this exercise has another bonus. There is an emerging field of research that looks at the effects of physical activity on our psychological fitness. *The Times* newspaper, not known for sensational headlines about health, recently declared that 'Exercise is essential to grow back your brain'. The report highlighted the work of a group of academics whose primary focus was on cardiovascular health. During the course of their research they discovered that those who had walked more had 'greater grey matter' in their brains and the 'greater grey matter volume reduced the risk for cognitive impairment twofold'. In layman's terms, physical activity had actually increased the amount of brain tissue, in the same way that physical activity can increase the amount of muscle tissue.

Professor Carol Brayne, who leads the research programme on 'Cognitive Function and Ageing' at the University of Cambridge, has concluded that 'even having a vigorous walk a few times a week' can lower the risk of dementia and Alzheimer's.

Bringing it all together

Let's recap what we've covered:

BE CONFIDENT OF THE BENEFITS OF FITNESS

Although fitness is usually associated with youth and gyms, it becomes more important the older you are. There is also good scientific evidence that fitness can be improved at any age – it's literally never too old to start.

THINK AND ACT EVERY DAY

There is an old Scottish proverb, which says, 'Many a mickle makes a muckle', i.e. many little things make a big thing. So if you bend your knees thirty times a day, that doesn't sound much, but thirty times a day = 10,950 times a year (and 10,980 in a leap year!).

It is very important, therefore, that unless you are acutely ill or recovering from an operation, you should do your daily ten minutes.

ALWAYS COVER ALL THE FOUR BIG Ss

Try and walk for thirty minutes every day – even if it's in ten minute slots – use the time for you – enjoy it! Get active – cycle three times a week if you can, and enjoy all the different activities there are out there, from swimming, bowls and dancing to tennis, cycling and skiing.

Stretch! Get supple with our suggested stretches.

Balance skills – improve your sense of balance to help avoid falls.

Strength – use your dumbbells and exercise band exercises to make your body more invincible.

Remember – a little change *every day* over a year really adds up. Think and act every day to improve your:

- **s**tamina

- **s**trength

- **s**kill (balance)

- **s**uppleness

All are equally important and all can be improved at any age.

IF YOU DO DEVELOP A DISEASE, ASK ABOUT EXERCISE

Almost every long-term condition benefits from fitness training but, with the exception of exercise therapists and physiotherapists, it is rarely mentioned when the prescription is handed over. So if you develop a problem, just ask the doctor about it. Tell them what you do already – for example 'I do 10 minutes exercise every day and try to fit four or five longer spells of walking or cycling into my life. There's no problem with that, is there?' It's highly unlikely that they'll say yes. Unfortunately, it is still rare for people to be given additional exercise related to the problem they are having with their shoulder, or their breathing, or their back, or whatever is the new problem. So you have to ASK.

So, we've covered the basics – you're geared up to stretch, improve your strength – now, get out there, get your heart rate up and start to deliver on your pledge to stand on one leg while you brush your teeth. You know you're doing the right thing!

3

THE ART OF BODY MAINTENANCE

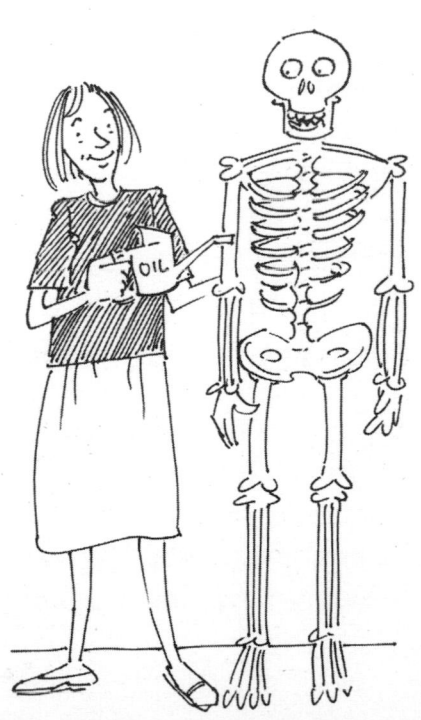

A 67-year-old friend has a 67-year-old car – a Morris Minor convertible. It is much admired, greatly loved and goes very nicely, although he would not set off to drive quickly to York or Land's End in it. It does require more care and maintenance than a Mini, the modern equivalent. The Morris Minor is a classic car, and you should care for your body like a classic car. You might not have the body of a 20-year-old person, but your body is a classic, and needs care and attention to keep it in the best possible condition!

You also need to keep an eye open for early signs of trouble. Regular servicing has become fashionable for cars, but it carries risks. The servicing of a car often results in extra expenditure and sometimes creates problems. So too can general health screening.

There is no need for you to have regular screening of your whole body, but one or two specific tests are recommended for all the parts of the body in the sections below. Remember – it's simpler than you think – most body maintenance, like the washing and polishing of your car, is best done by you.

New Year's resolutions

Happy New Year! This traditional greeting on the first of January is followed by the setting of New Year's resolutions, often to take more exercise or stop smoking. Many of these good intentions do not last until February, never mind change our lives. However, I want you to set and keep some resolutions as the result of reading this book, and I want you to keep them and to revisit them every year.

How do we make good resolutions – ones we can keep? Resolutions need to be:

- *specific* – focused on a clear area, such as losing weight or doing more exercise. What about something like 'I'm going to eat more healthily and lose weight'

- *measurable* – you need to keep a record and define your goals. For example, 'I'm going to lose enough weight to fit into my old jeans'

- *realistic* – it is all too easy to set unrealistic resolutions which cannot be achieved, creating a sense of failure. 'I'm going to be as slim as I was when I was a teenager by the end of this year' is something many of us are unlikely to achieve

- *shared* – tell other people about your resolutions so that they can support and encourage you.

Instead of simply thinking 'I must exercise more' or 'I must look after my teeth better', it is better to write down a resolution stating exactly what action you will take. Each of the sections below ends with suggestions of suitable resolutions. Make sure you keep the written resolution somewhere obvious – don't tuck it away in a drawer where it can be forgotten about. For example, your resolutions for maintaining the health of your teeth and gums (see page 123) could be stuck to the back of the bathroom cabinet door, next to the toothbrushes.

In this chapter we're going to go through parts of your body in turn. By the end you should know:

- the effects of the ageing process

- what you can do to compensate for these effects

- the early warning signs of serious disease.

The steps you take can have a massive impact on your health and help you avoid or postpone the onset of disease.

1. Brain maintenance

The brain and the mind are intimately inter-related, but we're going to look at them separately in this book because 'growing old' presents particular challenges to the mind *that have nothing to do with the brain*. The effects of ageing on the brain are very mild, but very common: principally problems with memory, reaction times and balance control. Although mood changes (especially depression) can be caused by brain diseases such as dementia, or by life circumstances related to ageing, depression is rarely a problem of the ageing process itself. Let's look at the brain first.

THE EFFECTS OF AGEING

Unlike most other tissues, such as the skin and the liver, brain cells cannot divide after birth. Therefore, while liver cells can increase if part of the liver is damaged or removed during an operation, brain cells cannot. Changes can be seen within and around the brain cells in everyone, and there are certain changes that are an inevitable result of ageing.

There is, as discussed in the chapter on fitness, some evidence that exercise can affect the tissue of the brain, but as yet there is no medical treatment that can stop or slow the changes in the brain.

At present, what *you* can do for your brain is more significant than what the medical profession can do.

WHAT YOU CAN DO

Remember the classic car? It needs more care than a new car. Your brain too now needs more care to be protected from preventable harm.

The first step is to ensure that the blood supply to the brain is as good as it can be, and this means taking the following precautions.

- *stop smoking*. Don't worry if you have tried unsuccessfully a dozen times before, just try again. There are numerous books detailing different methods of giving up; a good one is *The Only Way to Stop Smoking Permanently* by

Allen Carr. You should also have a look at the NHS's Smokefree web page at www.nhs.uk/smokefree

- *improve your metabolism.* The simplest way to do this is to lose weight. Aim for the weight you were at 30. See pages 80–1 for ideas for doing this

- *exercise.* Get walking! This helps by improving the function of the heart and lungs and helps you lose weight but it also has a direct beneficial effect on the brain tissue.

The second step is to protect your brain from the effects of chemicals – notably alcohol (on which subject see the section on digestion and the liver, page 73), but also some prescribed medication that can affect the way your brain functions. If you have concerns about your medication, discuss them with your pharmacist or doctor.

The third step is to improve your balance to prevent falling – many people suffer concussion following a fall in the home. Do the balance exercises on pages 47–9 and improve your chances of restabilising if you feel wobbly, and remember, most falls occur in the safety of your home!

The fourth step is to protect your brain while cycling or skiing. If you do indulge in these sports, always wear a helmet to avoid even slight knocks to the skull, in order to reduce the risk of concussion. If you do suffer a blow

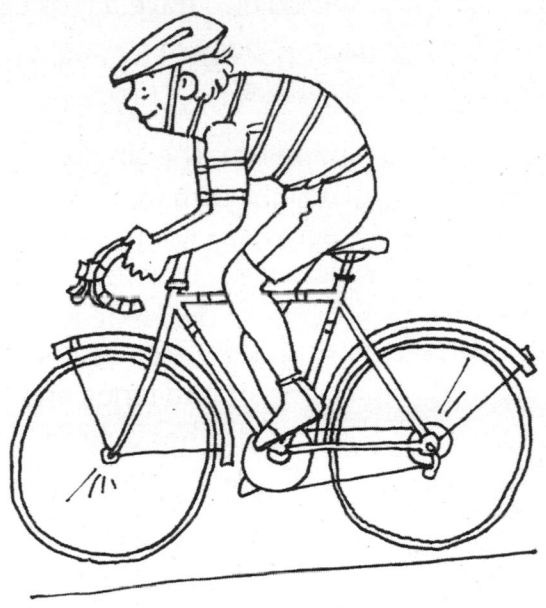

to your head, it is always best to seek medical attention, especially if you notice any symptoms (such as sickness) occurring as a result.

EARLY WARNING SIGNS

A sudden loss of intellectual ability, usually indicated by difficulty with speaking, may be a sign of stroke. A stroke is a major brain event. This simple FAST checklist summarises the symptoms to look out for either in yourself or in someone else:

- **F**ace drooping on one side – ask the person to smile to bring out the difference

- **A**rm weakness – ask the person to hold up both arms; watch to see if one drops down

- **S**peech difficulty – is the speech slurred or difficult to understand? Can the person repeat a simple sentence like 'the sky is blue'?

- **T**ime – call 999 as quickly as possible if any of these three things is occurring.

Although strokes can occur without these physical signs, a more common cause of a decline in reasoning or communication is depression, and this warning sign may be overlooked or attributed to 'dementia'. Persistent problems with memory or near misses when driving should be discussed with your doctor.

Resolution for better brain maintenance

Write down and stick to a resolution along these lines:

- every day I will do some exercise for the good of my brain as well as for physical fitness

- I will drink less and STOP SMOKING

- I will do the balance exercises to help avoid falls (see pages 47–9).

Let's now look at mind and memory maintenance.

2. Mind maintenance

The mind is related to the brain, but not in the simple way that muscles and joints are related to movement. Changes in the brain due to disease or ageing do affect the mind, but, as everyone knows, things go wrong with the mind even in people who have nothing wrong with their brain.

We can break down the mind's functions into two categories:

- cognitive – for example, memory, reasoning and logic

- emotional – for example, anxiety and depression

The two functions, cognitive and emotional, are interwoven, so that changes in one affect the other. In this section I'm going to concentrate on cognitive function and look at emotional issues in the chapter on wellbeing – see page 165.

THE EFFECTS OF AGEING

Some changes in memory, reasoning and decision-making are so common – indeed, may be regarded as universal – that many of us just assume they are the result of normal brain ageing. But research shows that *it is unlikely that these changes result solely from ageing*. A proportion of the problems that occur are due to environmental factors such as spending more time on your own because of a disabling disease affecting your ability to get out – not 'old age'. This is not to deny that some changes can cause problems.

Memory loss is experienced by almost all of us as we get older, particularly loss of short-term memory. While we are still able to remember much of what was learned in geography, English and chemistry fifty years before, or the names of the players in the football team of that era, recently acquired information is not so well retained – names, for example. It cannot be denied that this can be frustrating, but it is not a big problem and can be overcome.

On top of this, reasoning and decision-making processes are slower as a result of ageing. But again, *the actual size of the problem has been exaggerated*, as indeed have the benefits of quick decision-making. I think we should reframe this as a positive, and re-claim our right to make decisions more carefully!

OK, in certain situations (taking part in a quiz, for example), speed of thought is important, but most decisions, and certainly almost all serious decisions, do not need to be taken at speed. Young people who make decisions quickly may make the wrong decision! One reason for this, as outlined by Daniel Kahneman (winner of the Nobel Prize in Economics), is that people tend to think they are making decisions quickly and rationally when, in fact, the quick decision is often based on a rule of thumb that they have developed unconsciously and which leads them down the wrong path.

So it is not all about speed. The criticism that we older people are slow can be countered by saying that we are *reflective decision-makers*. Similarly, the criticism that old people are conservative can be countered by saying that we are not so rash.

WHAT YOU CAN DO

Get enough sleep

It is very important to get enough sleep, to reduce stress, and keep the mind working well. The amount of sleep that people need varies, but many of us need more sleep as we age. This need is often increased by the side effects of some of the medications that are commonly prescribed for blood pressure and heart disease for example. Here are some simple rules to help you get a good nights sleep:

- set a target, for example, seven hours a night

- don't nap in the daytime

- increase exercise during the day – WALK!

- learn the mindfulness technique (discussed on page 176) to stop ideas racing round your mind as you try to get off or if you wake in the middle of the night

- drink less fluid after 6 p.m. to avoid nightly trips to the loo.

- have a regular ritual for going to bed at the same time, with no exciting films or distressing news images beforehand, and choose a peaceful book

- stick to this better sleep programme!

Improve your memory

First, you can minimise or compensate for the loss of what is called 'short-term memory'. Here are some suggestions:

- ask people with uncommon names about the origin of their names; for example, 'Hussellbee? Where does that name come from?' Repeating the name back to someone might help you remember it.

- write down a person's email address. This can often be useful when you have been told someone's name but have forgotten it – many people's email addresses include their name in the firstname.lastname@gmail.com format.

A tactic similar to this was employed by a famous politician whose name, we shall say, was MacDonald. When he saw someone approaching who obviously expected to be recognised but whose name he had forgotten, he would alert his wife and then say, 'You haven't met my wife I think?' and she would then hold out her hand and say, 'I'm Nancy Smith', her maiden name, and this almost always nudged the other person into replying, 'Pleased to meet you, I'm Dudley Jones.'

There are many other techniques that can be used to compensate for the loss of short-term memory. Try these:

- write down appointments and details as soon as they are made – your smartphone offers an easy way to do this

- check your 'to do' list at the same time every day

- become more regular in your routine tasks – for example, always leave spectacles and keys in the same place.

Improve your reasoning

It is also essential to take steps to prevent the loss of the other cognitive functions, such as decision-making.

There is increasing evidence that the intellectual functions of the brain can be maintained by the equivalent of our body fitness training in chapter 2. In his book called *Smarter: the New Science of Building Brain Power*, the author Don Hurley tells us to have a daily brain 'workout':

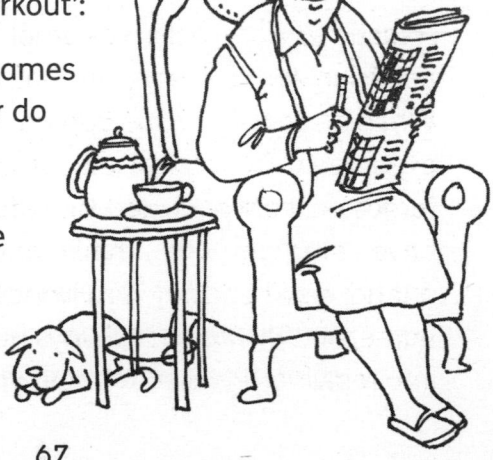

- play intellectual games such as Sudoku or do crosswords every day. As soon as you feel the game is becoming easy, either take up a new game or move up a league, for example, from simple crosswords to cryptic crosswords. *Cracking Cryptic Crosswords* by Colin Dexter, the creator of Inspector Morse, is an excellent book to help you make the transition from quick to cryptic crosswords

- learn something new, it doesn't matter what – it's all about avoiding standing still and letting your brains atrophy – keep challenging yourself! It doesn't have to be learning a new language in a week – it could be something like learning how to use a computer or researching your family history or how to Skype your grandchildren!

Get involved

As well as the steps you can take on your own, there is increasingly strong evidence that getting involved with other people maintains and improves intellectual functioning. The way it does this is not yet clear, but it may be the need to argue and defend a point of view as well as the need to use your mind. It may also be the interaction with other people that stimulates the mind, and that increased motivation and morale improves performance, in the same way that an athlete performs better in front of a crowd. Opportunities for this abound:

- work as a volunteer on an issue that you feel strongly about, either helping people less fortunate that yourself or protecting the environment. Age UK (www.ageuk.org.uk) is a great organisation with strong local branches with lots of opportunities both paid and unpaid. Supporting it and helping it support others will also help you

- work for income, particularly in jobs that younger people do not want to do. Much of the care for elderly people with frailty is provided by voluntary services run by people in their sixties and seventies. Now there is a new start-up company called Seniors Helping Seniors (www. seniorshelpingseniors.com), which specifically employs people who are older. It is right to be concerned about keeping young people out of employment but there are many jobs that older people are well suited for and which are unattractive to many younger people. The 'Age of No Retirement' is a campaign to encourage people to keep working.

- start a business – make things, sell things, do things

- enter politics, run for office in your area as a councillor, or volunteer as a school governor.

A major research study of ageing in Europe emphasised the importance of 'continued involvement in physical and social activities' for ageing well, and recommended that 'far from retiring, engagement with life and society should be the norm for ageing populations'. Many of us take a step back when we retire, not sure of our place in the community, and the transition from work to retirement can, of course, be difficult. But it's important to remember that as we move into our seventies we have a lot to offer – decades of understanding, experience and life knowledge – which will otherwise go to waste. And many of us have TIME – something the next generation often lack – share that time with them, offer to help wherever possible and you'll be surprised by how grateful people in your community will be!

So, make a vow to volunteer, get involved, get out there and use your considerable life knowledge to help those less experienced than you!

Resolution for better mind maintenance

Write down and stick to a resolution along these lines.

Every day I will:

- tax my brain at least three times a day either at work or by doing Sudoku or a crossword

- work on learning something new at least five days a week (for example, a musical instrument or a new language)

- get involved in my local community.

3. Digestive system and liver maintenance

It is quite amazing that our digestive system remains so healthy considering the stuff we put through it over the decades. The food we eat is the cause, wholly or partly, of many of our modern epidemics such as heart disease, Type 2 diabetes and some cancers, including bowel cancer. However, the gut and the liver remain relatively unscathed despite the fact that they transport many noxious chemicals from the outside world into our bloodstream.

THE EFFECTS OF AGEING

The gut may become less effective at digesting food and then absorbing the sugar, fat and protein molecules, but rarely does this cause problems in our seventies. For most of us, the gut remains pretty efficient. Many of us, however, do suffer from two particular problems in our seventies – constipation and irritable bowel syndrome (IBS). These often occur together because, although the main symptoms of IBS are pain, discomfort, bloating and frequent bowel motions, constipation can also be a feature. For others, however, the principal problem, is constipation.

It is now widely accepted that these conditions are not the consequences of ageing. They are the consequences of years, indeed decades, of consuming a diet with too little fibre. This could be regarded as a loss of fitness of the muscles in the intestine. The intestine, both large and small, is a muscular tube; the muscle tissue of the gut is different from the muscle tissue of the limbs, but the same principle holds true – if you don't use muscle, it becomes weak. Use it or lose it!

Similarly, most liver disease is caused not by ageing of the liver tissue but either by infection (hepatitis) or dietary factors. The latter notably include too much alcohol and too many calories with obesity now becoming a major cause of liver disease, so there is much that can be done, even if you start at 70.

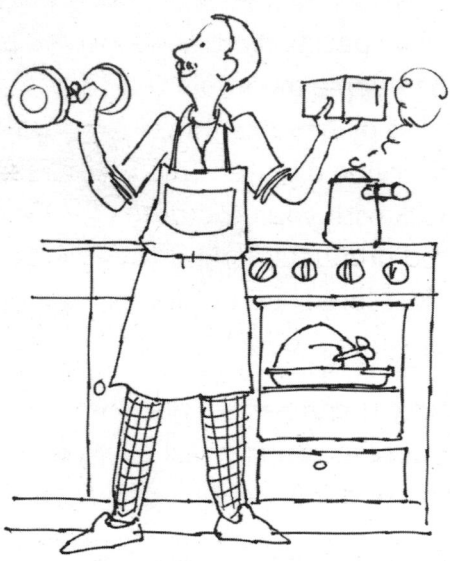

WHAT YOU CAN DO

Obviously 'eat less to prevent weight gain' is sound advice. But, so far as your digestive system is concerned, the key message, summed up in a *British Medical Journal* editorial in January 2014, is 'eat more fibre'. You need to eat a mixture of soluble and insoluble fibre.

Soluble fibre foods include oats, nuts, seeds, beans, lentils and most fruits. Insoluble fibre is found in wheat bran, most vegetables, and whole grains such as barley, bulgur wheat, millet, brown rice, rye, oats and whole wheat. Eat fruit and vegetables every day, as in the five-a-day rule. Try eating fish and chicken more often than red meat. Try to incorporate as many of these foods into your diet as possible – even small changes like switching from white bread to whole grain can make a difference.

Be aware of any specific dietary needs you might develop. Some people are intolerant to gluten, and if you are troubled by Irritable Bowel Syndrome (IBS) it may be worth trying a gluten-free diet to see if that has an effect (check with your doctor first). Gluten is found in wheat based products and has been linked to bowel discomfort. Most large supermarkets now stock a good range of gluten-free products.

So far as alcohol is concerned, there is no need to stop completely, but research suggests that from the age of 70 you should not drink:

- more than four days a week; and

- on the days you drink alcohol don't drink more than three units of alcohol a day for men, two units if you are a woman.

To help you calculate the units, one unit is:

- a small glasses of wine

- a half pint of beer
- a single shot of spirits.

Cutting down on alcohol also helps with your weight because alcohol is rich in calories, not very filling and often increases appetite – a triple whammy. You need to be careful also that your alcohol intake does not creep up due to lower cost alcohol, combined with the subtle effect of bigger wine glasses (two glasses of wine these days can often empty an entire bottle!) and the fact that you don't need to get up and out early for work the next morning. Why not have three or four days without alcohol every week? If you want to see an excellent alcohol unit calculator, go to the NHS website at www.nhs.uk and put 'sensible drinking' into the search box. Be honest with your answers to the questions.

Remember that if you are still working or want to use your brain in the afternoon, alcohol at lunchtime should be avoided completely.

EARLY WARNING SIGNS

Passing blood in your bowel motions or sudden alteration in bowel habit, either diarrhoea or constipation, that persists for more than three weeks, or abdominal pain, may be symptoms of bowel cancer and you should consult your doctor. Pain in the lower left part of the abdomen can be caused by something called diverticulitis which may be considered as a complication of long term Irritable Bowel Syndrome. This can lead to the creation of little bulges through the muscular wall of the colon which can become infected. This is not a forerunner of cancer but recurrent pain should be reported to your doctor. There is another more serious condition called Inflammatory Bowel Disease, confusingly called IBD, and formerly known as ulcerative colitis, which also causes pain, diarrhoea and bleeding. Always take anal bleeding seriously and go and see your doctor immediately.

Resolution for better digestive system and liver maintenance

Write down and stick to a resolution along these lines.

I will:

- eat more fibre

- eat fruit and vegetables at least five times a day

- eat fish and chicken more often than red meat

- not drink more than the recommended limit more than once a month

- have three days without any alcohol each week.

4. Metabolic maintenance

The metabolic system provides the body's energy using food and oxygen. The metabolic rate – the rate at which energy is produced and used – is controlled not only by the way you live your life, but also by hormones which are produced by another system – the endocrine system. This is the system of glands such as the thyroid and the pancreas.

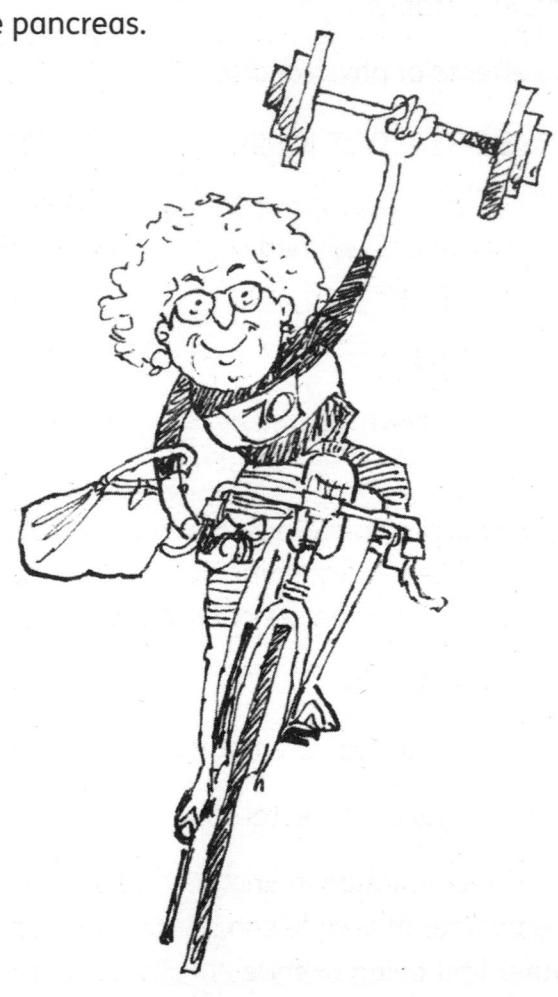

THE EFFECTS OF AGEING

The metabolic rate slows a little as we grow older, but there are two important points to remember.

First, this does not mean that it is inevitable that you will slow down as you get older. Many of us notice a loss of energy as we get older, but this is principally due to other factors, notably:

- the effects of physical disease
- the effects of psychological problems such as depression
- the side-effects of medication for physical or mental disease
- loss of fitness.

And, of course, more than one of these factors is often present.

The main metabolic problem that affects people in their sixties and seventies, sometimes called metabolic syndrome, has a common set of features:

- being overweight
- a diagnosis of Type 2 diabetes
- raised levels of cholesterol.

Surveys of the population in England indicate that about one quarter of people can be classified as obese with another half being overweight. These factors can raise the risk of heart disease, stroke and cancer. However, it is important to see these conditions not so much as diseases in their own right, but as an inevitable result of years or decades of us consuming more calories than we need.

Weight gain, metabolic syndrome and Type 2 diabetes result from the decrease in energy expenditure that affects most people from the age of 20. This does not mean that they are due to decrease in sweaty exercise in lycra and a gym; primarily, they are likely to be caused by a decrease in walking. Metabolic syndrome and Type 2 diabetes are often portrayed as being due to the consumption of too many calories, and it is true that this is a factor in some people. However, the basic cause is not due to surplus but to deficiency. They can be regarded as consequences of one of the epidemics of modern life – the *walking deficiency syndrome*.

The epidemic of Type 2 diabetes is the direct result of the epidemic of inactivity, the effects of which have built up over decades of a lifestyle in which the daily expenditure of energy was even 50 calories less than the intake because:

> 50 calories a day = 18,250 calories or five pounds of fat a year

It is a bit like Mr Micawber in *David Copperfield*, except in reverse. So far as money is concerned, he said:

Income twenty shillings, expenditure nineteen and six, result happiness.

Income twenty shillings, expenditure twenty shillings and sixpence, result misery.

But so far as health is concerned:

Energy intake 2,000 calories daily, expenditure 1,900 calories, result ... metabolic syndrome and unhappiness.

WHAT YOU CAN DO – LOSING WEIGHT

Even in our own time the amount of energy expended at work or in the home has steadily reduced, and mercifully so. No one wants to go back to the world before washing machines or fork lift trucks, but we do have to recognise that we live in a different environment, one that is full of new risks. The risks of industrial accidents and disease have been dramatically reduced, but they have been replaced by the risks of inactivity due to changes in work and at home, and the principal villain is the car!

There is much hand-wringing in the press about the modern diet and its contribution to an 'epidemic of obesity', but there is a growing consensus that the change that correlates most closely with the increase in obesity is not diet but the increase in car ownership.

For people aged 70, the growing availability of, and reliance on, the car has reduced the amount of energy we spend on getting to work, shopping and recreation. Many people would use as much energy if they simply walked to and from the gym or leisure centre rather than driving there and back, and that includes the energy used in the exercise session.

More walking, combined with a better diet, is a really effective way of preventing, treating and curing the metabolic syndrome and Type 2 diabetes.

Losing weight

Your weight may have increased between the ages of 60 and 70. Some people are lucky and experience a welcome reduction in weight after retirement as a consequence of less sitting at a desk or in a car. Remember your weight at the age of 30 and aim for that as your target. To reach the target you need to:

- Change your diet by eating –

    » more vegetables

    » more fruit (at least five helpings of fruit and vegetables a day)

    » more fibre (both soluble and insoluble)

    » fish and chicken instead of red meat

    » olive oil instead of butter and lard

» less sugar – biscuits, cake, sweeties, chocolate and sugar in any form

- Increase the amount of exercise you take – thirty minutes walking every day for a year is equivalent to ten pounds of fat!

Your healthier eating programme

The word 'diet' is a funny one. Originally, in the Middle Ages, it meant, according to that wonderful book, the *Shorter Oxford English Dictionary*, 'to prescribe or regulate the food of a person.' Then a little later, in 1660 to be precise, a new meaning was developed 'to regulate oneself as to diet' and both these meanings survive today. However, in the 21st century the word has come to be associated only with weight loss and with eating less. The scientific evidence is certainly that many people, perhaps more than half the people in the UK aged 70 and over, would improve their health if they lost weight, and their joints would heave a sigh of relief too. To know whether or not to lose weight, look in a mirror and BE HONEST!

A good diet for people in their seventies certainly requires less of some foodstuffs, but it also requires an increase in others. A good diet for people in the developed countries means both less and more.

Eat (and Drink) Less	Eat (and Drink) More
Sugar, including biscuits, chocolate and sweets	Vegetables – and try to grow some of them if you can
Cakes	Fruit, go for at least five helpings of fruit or vegetables a day
Red meat	Fish
Sausages and processed meats like salami and ham	Chicken
Fried food	Steamed food
Butter and cream	Olive oil
Full cream milk	Semi-skimmed or skimmed milk, to keep up your calcium
Alcoholic and sweet drinks – alcoholic drinks are very high in calories	Water
Low fibre food such as white bread and white flour	High fibre food, brown or wholemeal bread, wholemeal flour and high fibre grain such as brown rice, millet, bulgur wheat and oats If you can see the content of bread, look for breads that have *less than* 10 grams of carbohydrate to one gram of fibre. If you can see the content of cereals that have *less than* five grams of carbohydrate to one gram of fibre

Remember too that eating 'well' is as important as good food. People in countries in which obesity is common often eat while watching television, with the result that when the plate is empty the person looks down and still feels hungry because their brain has not registered the fact that they have been eating. A.A. Gill, the well-known *Sunday Times* food critic writes that no-one should ever eat while walking because it reduces the awareness of the goodness of the food. Our parents' generation was influenced by Horace Fletcher's principle that every mouthful should be chewed thirty-two times. This practice, called Fletcherism, can help not only your digestion but also with your weight control by helping you feel fuller because you are concentrating more on the act of eating.

Remember that exercise is the other side of the weight loss coin, so always think of food and exercise together. A healthier diet should be combined with my walking programme (see page 25) if you are keen to lose weight.

EARLY WARNING SIGNS

Early warning signs of Type 2 diabetes may be tiredness and thirst, and you should report these symptoms to the doctor. But it is also advisable to look at yourself in the mirror regularly. If your body shape has changed significantly since you were 30 – *be honest* about it – then go and see the doctor.

Sudden loss of weight that is unplanned is a change that should be reported to your doctor. Increase in weight combined with tiredness that occurs

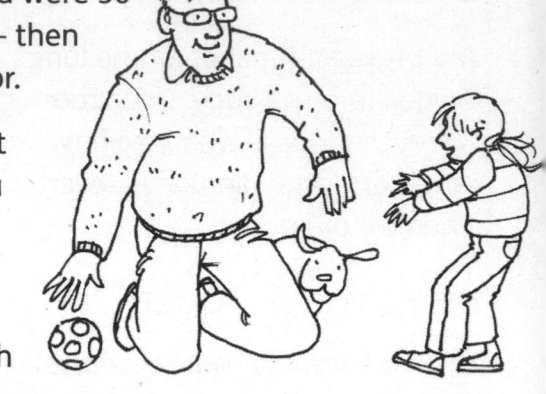

over a year may also indicate a thyroid disorder, so also visit your doctor if you have noticed these symptoms. Obesity is increasing in all age groups, most worryingly in children, so when the grandchildren come over give them an activity not sweets!

Resolution for better metabolic maintenance

Write down and stick to a resolution along these lines.

I will:

- adjust my diet and my activity to reduce my weight to the weight I was at 30

- take thirty minutes extra exercise at least three times a week

- eat more fibre every day.

5. Lung maintenance

The principal function of the lungs is to get enough oxygen into the body. If function is impaired, the result is breathlessness when we have to exert ourselves. However, if the damage is severe, this will occur even when we are at rest.

THE EFFECTS OF AGEING

The world record by a 70-year-old man for running one mile is 5 minutes 19 seconds, set by Joop Ruter in 2003. The record for cycling 25 miles, as set by John Woodburn when aged 71, is 54 minutes 21 seconds, the equivalent of 27.7mph. The effects of ageing alone on the lung are obviously relatively unimportant because this level of performance, which very few people aged 20 could achieve, is enabled by a pair of lungs that have aged for fifty years. For most of us, however, our lung function at the age of 70 has been affected by a number of other factors:

- the Clean Air Act was passed in 1956. Therefore, someone aged 70 in 2014 spent the first twelve years of their life if they lived in a city in an environment that caused severe damage to their growing lungs. Remember those filthy black fogs?

- The first *Report on Smoking and Health* was published by the Royal College of Physicians in 1962. When we were teenagers, smoking was very prevalent and acceptable, with the result that the lungs of many people in their seventies were damaged by their parents' smoking, or their own smoking, or both.

Furthermore, the body's ability to use oxygen is determined not only by lung function but also by the ability of muscle cells to extract oxygen from the bloodstream. As fitness is lost, this ability deteriorates too, so any increase in breathlessness is, like many other changes, blamed on ageing, whereas it is, in fact, due to both environmental factors and loss of fitness.

The good news is that it is possible to slow down the rate of developing breathlessness and even improve our body's ability to get enough oxygen.

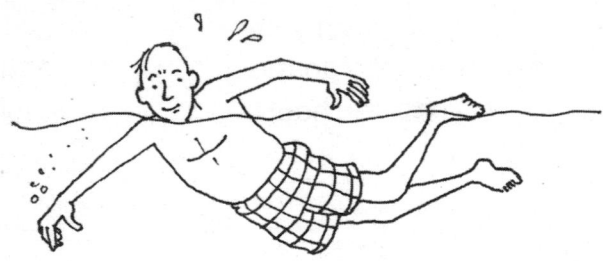

WHAT YOU CAN DO

- If you smoke, try to stop, now, immediately (see the box, on stopping smoking opposite)

- Make sure you get your influenza and pneumococcal pneumonia vaccines (see page 147).

- Take exercise that makes you breathless at least three days a week. Heavy housework, cycling, dancing, swimming and brisk walking are examples of good exercise. It is the intensity of exercise that is important rather than the duration. It is better to do exercise that makes you so breathless that it affects the flow of conversation for ten minutes than to take a gentle stroll for thirty minutes. The main benefit of such exercise, which will improve your stamina, is not on the lungs but on the muscles. Within the muscles there are processes that extract oxygen from the blood as it passes through the muscle. These processes become more effective if they are stimulated by being forced to extract more oxygen regularly by working the muscles.

As always, taking action in your seventies will not only help you feel better, and do more; it will also reduce the risk that you will become housebound in your eighties and nineties. Jam today and tomorrow!

Your quit smoking programme

Stopping smoking in your seventies is still one of the best things you can do to improve your health, your attractiveness and your wellbeing in your eighties and nineties.

If you stop smoking at 70:

- the risk of getting lung cancer will stay stable and will not increase year on year, as it will if you carry on

---

- the risk of getting heart disease will reduce, and by the age of 80 will be the same as if you had never smoked

- the risks of having an anaesthetic if you have surgery will reduce

- symptoms of bronchitis will reduce

It is never too late to benefit from stopping smoking. Even if you have tried ten times before, try again, because there are now many more ways to help and support you.

Choose a good time to quit

Of course, any time is a good time but you can increase your chances of success by choosing a time which will motivate you, for example:

- your birthday

- New Year's Day

- when a grandchild is born, because you don't want to harm the baby with your second-hand smoke

Seek help from your GP or practice nurse

No matter how busy they are, they know that helping you to quit smoking is one of the best health services they can offer. They can simply refer you to a NHS stop smoking adviser. You can, of course, find a stop smoking adviser yourself and make direct contact; simply type your postcode into the smoke free webpage of NHS Choices www.nhs.uk/smokefree

Get support

The stop smoking adviser will give you support, but so too will friends and family. Some people find it hopeful to make a pledge to a charity for example, and ask friends to phone them daily for support. Your NHS Stop Smoking Service will also support you face-to-face and you can get daily emails and texts by enrolling either with an adviser or on the smoke free website.

Don't be afraid to try stop smoking medicines

One reason why people don't manage to quit is the distressing effects of nicotine withdrawal. But don't try to compensate by switching to e-cigarettes, ask for the drugs specifically designed to help cope with nicotine withdrawal symptoms. There are three types of stop smoking medicines:

- Champix tablets (vasenidine)

- Zyban tablets (bupropion)

- Nicotine Replacement Therapy, which is available as gum lozenges, nasal sprays, inhalers and patches.

If you still smoke, quit. If you have tried before, try again with support. If you have a friend who smokes, help them decide to quit and then quit together.

EARLY WARNING SIGNS

A new, persistent cough or hoarseness that lasts three weeks or more, or blood in your saliva, may be a sign of disease and you should consult your GP.

Resolution for better lung maintenance

Write down and stick to a resolution along these lines.

I will:

- take exercise that makes me breathless for ten minutes at least three times a week (brisk walking will do)

- get a flu shot every winter

- check whether my doctor thinks I need a pneumonia shot

- if you still smoke, *stop!*

6. Heart maintenance

We have seen a dramatic fall in the number of people dying or suffering from heart disease in the last twenty years. This is because of better prevention techniques and better treatment particularly of coronary heart disease – a blockage of the small arteries supplying the heart muscle itself. The heart is a big muscle and, like all muscles, is affected by ageing.

THE EFFECTS OF AGEING

As in all muscle tissue, the ageing process leads to a loss of power. Furthermore, the electrical impulses that cause the heart to beat change with age. The maximum rate at which the heart can beat decreases at about one per cent every year, but the effect of this would only be felt when people were exercising at their absolute limits, something we do not advise! However, most of the limitations that people experience, from heart failure to chest pain or an irregular pulse, are not caused by ageing, but by disease. One principal cause, again, is cigarette smoking. The Western diet is also known to increase the risk of heart disease, with the notable exception of the Mediterranean diet. Some of the loss of cardiac function is also due to loss of cardiac fitness, but that can be improved all the way through your seventies.

WHAT YOU CAN DO

There is much that you can do to prevent further decline in function due to loss of fitness and disease, even if you already have heart disease:

- first, if you smoke, stop (see page 87)

- second, take exercise that will increase your pulse rate, at least three days a week. Remember, this does not require going to the gym or wearing lycra! Brisk walking, cycling, dancing or swimming will all achieve this level of activity

- adapt your diet to the healthier option (see page 82)

- make sure your blood pressure is not high and take action to reduce it if it is, namely by:

  » losing weight (see page 99)

  » taking blood pressure medicine to lower it if it has been prescribed.

There is much debate about the part that drugs like statins can play in preventing heart disease in people who have never had any symptoms. At present statins are not prescribed for people at very low risk; but some people are now taking the polypill, a pill that combines a number of different drugs but at lower doses than those prescribed by doctors. The polypill has been developed to give people at low risk an opportunity of reducing their risk even further, with a reduced risk of side-effects.

If you already have heart disease, or disease of the heart and blood vessels, the importance of improving cardiac fitness and reducing the risk of further deterioration and heart attacks is even more important and just as achievable. If you have heart disease, like me, do everything that is recommended above, as well as undergoing the treatment recommended by your clinical advisers.

As with the lung maintenance programme (see page 85), some of the benefit of taking exercise to improve the heart's function also helps in other parts of the body too. For example, intermittent claudication, (derived from the Latin word for limping) is a condition where people (usually men who have smoked) have to stop frequently because of pain in their leg muscles due to insufficient oxygen. The effects of exercise combined with the right medical treatment will not only improve cardiac output but also make the muscles more effective at extracting oxygen from the blood passing through them, often preventing the need for an operation to replace the narrowed artery.

You should also seriously consider the offers made to everyone by the NHS:

- to have a health check

- to be screened for abdominal aortic aneurysm, a swelling of the major artery (the aorta), as it runs through the abdominal cavity. This offer is made only to men because the condition is very uncommon in women.

EARLY WARNING SIGNS

Chest pain or a sudden increase in breathlessness, either during exercise or while at rest, is a symptom that should not be ignored. Call an ambulance or get someone to drive you to the A&E department of a hospital.

Resolution for better heart maintenance

Write down and stick to a resolution along these lines.

I will:

- change my diet to a healthier option (see page 82)

- take exercise that makes me breathless for at least ten minutes at least three days a week – brisk walking will do

- take any medication that has been prescribed to reduce the risk of heart disease regularly.

7. Muscle maintenance

'Use it or lose it' is a piece of advice now widely known and used, for example, when the future of a local library is being discussed; however, it was first used with regard to muscle. If you don't use your muscles, they will waste away and as we have already discussed, research has revealed that much of the loss of muscle tissue which we have assumed was an inevitable consequence of ageing is, in fact, the result of inactivity. In the 1980s one of my colleagues, Archie Young, a doctor with a special interest in exercise and later Professor of Geriatrics in Edinburgh, took muscle cells from volunteers in his research project. The results convinced me how much the loss of power was due to inactivity rather than ageing. This does not mean the result of laziness, but a consequence of twentieth-century (and now twenty-first-century) life. The twentieth century was one in which the most important part of the anatomy was not the strong right arm or the sturdy legs but the bottom – it was the sitting century. An aggravating factor is that we're still told that those of us with chronic conditions should 'take it easy', whereas, in fact, we need to think even more about fitness.

THE EFFECTS OF AGEING

Ageing does affect muscle fibres. There are a number of changes that take place as we get older that reduce their power. And, the older we are, the quicker our muscle tissue is affected by inactivity. In men this may be aggravated by a decrease in testosterone. However, for many of us the principal cause of loss of muscle power is inactivity.

WHAT YOU CAN DO

Immediately start thinking about strength. While walking and running are important contributors for improving the strength of your leg muscles, there are many other muscles that need to be strengthened, particularly the muscles of the upper limbs and what are called the core muscles – abdomen, back and spine.

Carry out the strength training exercises outlined on page 29.

EARLY WARNING SIGNS

Muscles are rarely affected by serious disease. If an acute pain occurs during an excercise, you may have torn some muscle fibres. Simply apply an ice pack wrapped in a tea towel to the area (keep a bag of peas in the freezer for this purpose) and stop that particular exercise for two weeks.

If you have recently started a new drug, muscle pain may be a side effect and you should discuss this with your pharmacist, doctor or practice nurse. Statins are a type of drug which may cause this. Pain when walking in one or both calf muscles, usually coming on after the same distance, can be a symptom of a narrowing of the blood vessels in the leg and should be discussed with your doctor.

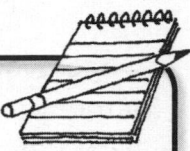

Resolution for better muscle maintenance

Write down and stick to a resolution along these lines.

I will:

- do strengthening exercises for the upper limbs every day. See page 38

- do strengthening exercises for the core muscles every day. See page 42.

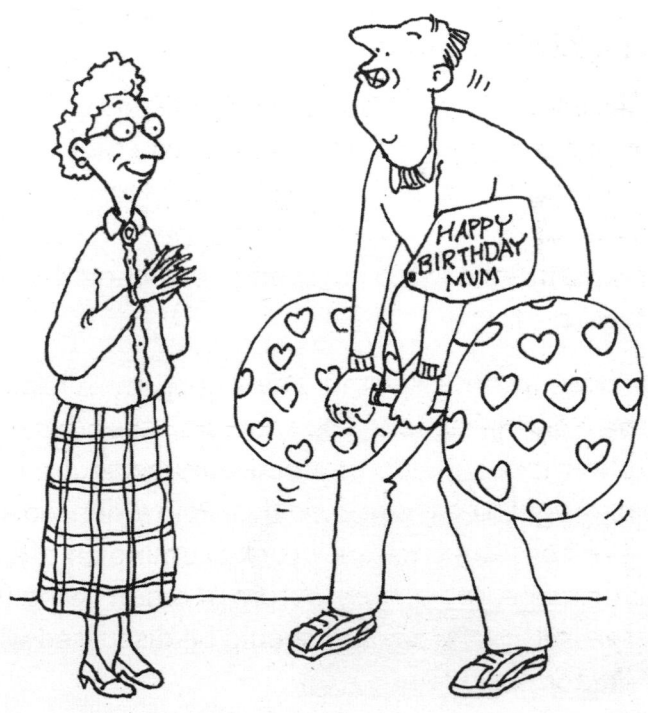

8. Bone maintenance

Although your skeleton is invisible, it is important to keep it strong. In fact, the older you get the stronger it needs to be to help reduce the risk of fractures. Your skeleton consists of bones, linked by joints. We will consider joint maintenance, including the bones of your spine, separately.

THE EFFECTS OF AGEING

Loss of tissue occurs as part of the ageing process. The terms 'osteopenia' and 'osteoporosis' are often used to describe this process, and they simply mean 'thinner bone' and 'much thinner bone'. These are not distinct diseases, however, they are serious conditions as, with age, everyone's bone tissue thins, increasing the risk of fractures. The strength of your bones at the age of 70 is determined by two factors:

- how strong your bones were at the age of 30

- how quickly you have been losing bone tissue.

You can obviously do nothing about the first of these factors, but you can slow the rate of bone loss through your seventies because, as is the case with most other age-related changes, it is determined not only by the ageing process alone but also by inactivity. The bone of even a young person becomes thinner if immobilised in a plaster cast, and one of the consequences of our less active lifestyle, and higher car ownership, is inactivity leading to loss of bone tissue.

WHAT YOU CAN DO

There are three things you can do to slow the rate of bone thinning:

- increase the amount of activity that puts pressure on your bones – the exercises recommended for increasing your muscular strength (see chapter 2) will also increase the strength of your bones

- take exercise – even a brisk walk strengthens the bones in your legs as a result of the impact of walking

- vitamin D is essential not only to prevent rickets in children but also to prevent bone weakening in your seventies. This is particularly important for women. Furthermore, it's important for everyone living in the UK, as the sun from October to April is not strong enough for us to produce vitamin D in our skin. Everyone is vitamin D deficient during the winter, as vitamin D can only be stored in the body for about six weeks. Vitamin D helps reduce falls by keeping muscles in better condition too. There is some evidence that it also reduces the risk of dementia

- the human skeleton needs about 1200mg dietary calcium per day to maintain the strength of the bones. Many people try to cut down on dairy products to reduce their cholesterol, and become calcium deficient as a result! You may know that skimmed milk has the least fat, but did you know that it also has the most calcium? Aim to have three or four portions of calcium-rich foods, such as milk, yoghurt, hard cheeses, sardines or even white bread. You can access calcium calculators online, but remember, the best way of getting calcium is through a healthy diet.

People who have been diagnosed with osteoporosis may be prescribed treatments such as additional calcium, however, everyone should consider taking vitamin D – 15–25mg a day. You can buy this supplement over the counter at a chemist or a large supermarket. If you have had a fracture caused in part by thin bones (for example, a wrist fracture), it is essential that you have medication to reduce the risk of a second 'fragility' fracture. If you are at risk of osteoparosis, you can ask for a 'Dual Energy Xray Absorptiometry' (DEXA) test to measure your bone density.

To reduce the risk of fractures you need to keep your bones as strong as possible and also reduce the risk of falling. Most falls occur at home, not outside, and they occur not so much because of loose rugs or slippery floors but because there is a momentary loss of balance from which you cannot recover without falling. This is often because the organs of balance become less effective as a result of ageing. However, you can reduce the risk of falling by doing exercises to keep strong and skilful, and there are exercises that specifically help you maintain and improve your ability to balance and to recover your position if you do stumble or trip (see page 47). Regular T'ai Chi has been shown to help reduce falls. You don't have to get up at dawn and stand in a meadow to do t'ai chi: there are good exercise DVDs you can work with in the privacy of your own home!

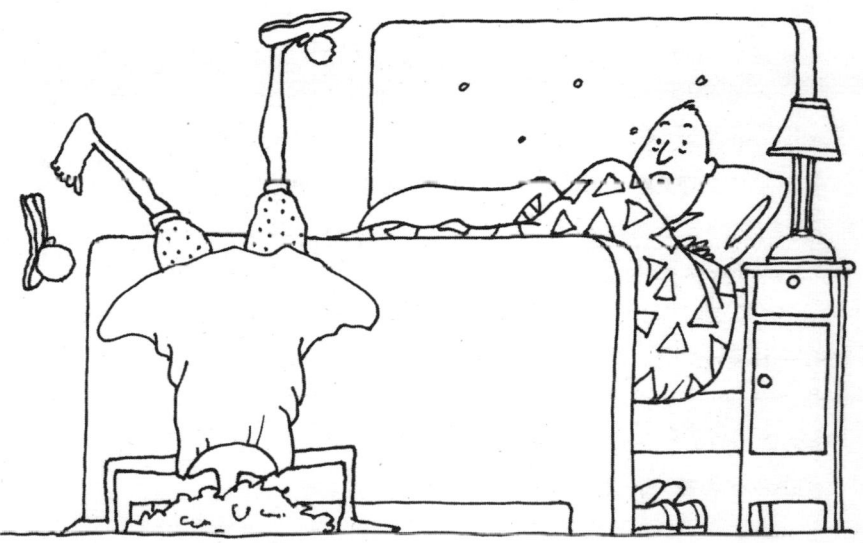

The National Osteoporosis Society produces excellent advice about maintaining bone health throughout your life. It recommends:

- exercise of all sorts including exercises that increase strength

- a healthy diet

- stopping smoking

- cutting back on alcohol, which helps the bones as well as the liver.

Of all the vitamins promoted and sold, vitamin D, 15–25mg a day, is the one that most people in relatively sunless northern countries should take. If you have been told you have thin bones, you should take the recommended dose of calcium too – although most people get enough calcium from their diet, principally from cheese and milk.

Resolution for better bone maintenance

Write down and stick to a resolution along these lines.

I will:

- keep to my strengthening exercises daily

- take other exercise, such as walking

- drink less

- stop smoking

- if I have decided to take 15 or 25 micrograms of vitamin D, take it every day.

9. Joint maintenance

For most of us, problems with joints are greater than problems with the bones themselves. Where two bones meet in a joint, the surface of each is covered by a hard, smooth, low-friction material called cartilage. The joint also has a small amount of lubricant called synovial fluid, contained by the 'joint capsule' (fibrous tissue that provides a sleeve attached to the bone on each side of the joint). Attached to (or near) the capsule are the ligaments and the tendons of muscles that move the joint and help keep it steady.

THE EFFECTS OF AGEING

Our cartilage thins with age, faster in some of us than in others, but there is no evidence that walking or cycling or moving the joints within their usual range wears out the cartilage and causes arthritis. Professional athletes do have more joint problems, but that is because they are using their joints in an abnormal way – for example, in the front row of a rugby scrum, they damage the capsule and ligaments. The fibrous tissue in tendons and ligaments loses elasticity as a result of ageing, but much of the stiffness that develops is not the result of ageing but due to loss of suppleness, which you can prevent.

WHAT YOU CAN DO

Loss of suppleness is less recognised by the fitness industry than loss of strength and stamina, but it is possible to improve your suppleness at any age and prevent further loss by the daily suppleness programme (see page 32).

It is also essential to keep the muscles around joints strong because the muscles support the joint. A vicious cycle can develop, as shown below.

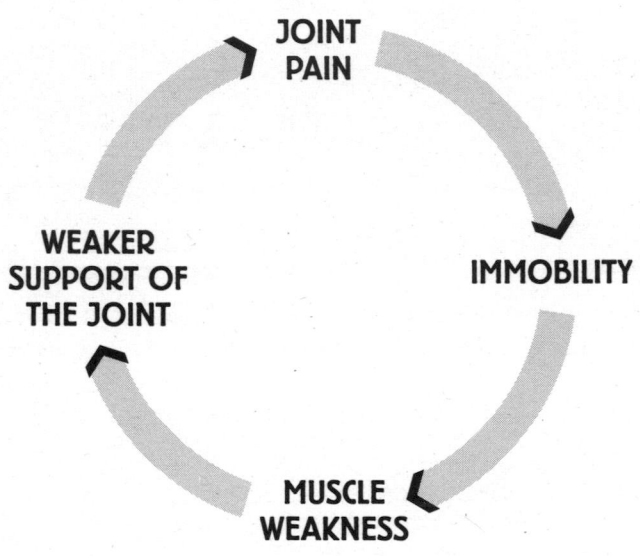

**How joint disease can get worse
due to the immobility it causes**

For the knees, your quadriceps muscles at the front of your thigh are of particular importance. For the hip, the gluteal or buttock muscles must be kept strong. Cycling helps both groups of muscles, but all activity is helpful, including dancing.

EARLY WARNING SIGNS

Stiffness and pain are the symptoms of joint disease. When they affect a single joint (the knee or the shoulder, for example), the condition is called osteoarthritis. The medical treatment for this consists of pain control and, for some people, joint replacement. However, many doctors themselves use a third 'treatment' – improving their suppleness to postpone the need for joint replacement surgery as long as possible. Hip and knee replacements are wonderful operations; the shoulder joint replacement is less well established. However, a proportion of operations do go wrong, even in the best orthopaedic hospitals, so most doctors keep going as long as they can with painkillers and suppleness exercises until they feel they really need the operation.

Pain that occurs in more than one joint, sometimes called 'polyarthritis', is usually caused by inflammation, with rheumatoid arthritis being the commonest diagnosis. But if muscles are painful too, the term 'polymyalgia rheumatica' is sometimes used and you should consult your GP if you are worried about this. Early morning pains, particularly in women, are a symptom of polymyalgia or rheumatoid arthritis.

Unfortunately, there are few early warning signs of osteoarthritis – everyone is at risk. If you have localised pain in any bone, go and see your doctor.

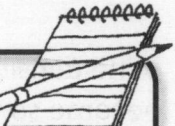

Resolution for better joint maintenance

Write down and stick to a resolution along these lines.

I will:

- keep to my strengthening exercises daily (see chapter 2)

- keep to my suppleness exercises daily (see page 32)

- not increase my weight from today and, if necessary, decrease it by keeping diet and exercise resolutions.

10. Spine maintenance

'*Somdel stope in age*' was Chaucer's description of an old person, and stooping is characteristic of many people in their seventies; again this is rarely the effect of ageing.

THE EFFECTS OF AGEING

The spine consists of a column of bones connected by complicated joints. So, like all bones and joints, there are changes that result from the ageing process.

The bones become thinner, but this rarely causes problems. For some of us, particularly women whose bone density was low at the age of 30, the bone may become so thin by the time they reach 70 – a condition called osteoporosis – that one or more vertebrae may fracture and collapse. There are many treatments that can help with this and prevent further fractures, so see your doctor if you experience any symptoms such as those mentioned in the early warning signs (see page 109).

The common loss of height that many people notice as they reach their seventies and eighties is usually caused by shrinkage of the discs between the vertebrae and changes in posture brought about by weakening of the back muscles. The joints between the vertebrae are also affected by ageing, but this too is not a cause of major problems.

Most of the problems of the spinal column are actually caused by preventable changes in the muscles and ligaments of the spinal column.

WHAT YOU CAN DO

Our spine is designed to carry the skull and the limbs in three beautiful curves:

- cervical spine – the neck – curving forward
- thoracic spine – the chest – curving backward
- lumbar spine – the lower back – curving forward

Unfortunately for many of us, years – indeed decades – of our life are spent with the spine in a single ugly curve with the head poking forward.

Driving or typing or sitting in meetings or lounging on a sofa all lead to the stooping spine, with head forward like a tortoise, not erect like a gazelle. Obviously this is hard to correct if it has been going on for decades (sadly, many teenagers slouch, but don't waste your energy telling them not to!). However, from the age of 70 you can take corrective action.

- if you can afford it, go to a Pilates or Alexander Technique class. If you cannot afford it, look for videos on Pilates and the Alexander Technique on Google

- adjust your car seat so that you sit straight, head *against* the headrest, with a small cushion behind your lumbar spine (lower back) if required.

- if you work at a desk, find a surface of the right height and work at your keyboard standing up. Find a little box to put one foot on and change from leg to leg. The motto is 'down with chairs, up with standing'

- find a set of stretching exercises from a teacher or the web that suits you and do them for at least five minutes every day. The starfish is particularly good:

» lie flat on your back on the floor

» stretch your arms out sideways, elbows on the carpet

» see if you can put the back of your hands on the carpet

» hold for ten seconds then repeat at least five times.

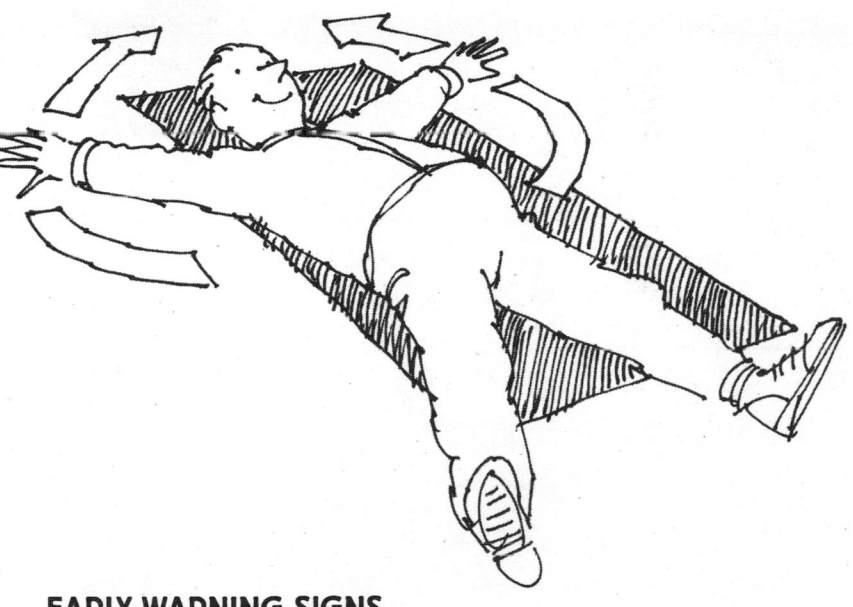

EARLY WARNING SIGNS

You may not notice any particular warning signs until you suffer a fragility fracture of the wrist, hip or a rib, but if you find yourself stooping or losing height then seek medical advice. If you experience acute pain in the spine itself, such as you have never had before, make an appointment with your GP.

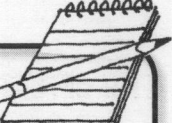

Resolution for better spine maintenance

Write down and stick to a resolution along these lines.

I will:

- do some kind of spinal stretching exercise every day – see page 42

- go for T'ai Chi, Alexander Technique or Pilates lessons at least once a year (suggest these courses if asked what you'd like for your birthday or Christmas)

- think, at least three times a day when standing or sitting, 'Is my posture good or am I stooping and peering forwards?'

11. Foot maintenance

A hand surgeon is of higher social standing than a podiatrist, reflecting the fact that hands are highly admired whereas our feet stay hidden. They just have to put up with being stood on for seventy years. Yet in your seventies and eighties, your feet are at least as important as your hands, unless you play the piano or violin. They need lots of care and attention.

THE EFFECTS OF AGEING

The foot is one of the architectural wonders of the body. Bones, joints, muscles, ligaments and tendons all fit together in perfect harmony, at least for the first ten years of life. For men's feet the next sixty years are pretty uneventful, except for the fact that each foot hits the ground about three and a half million times a year. Women's feet, however, face a few challenging decades as they are so often squeezed, forced or rammed into high-heeled shoes with pointed toes. This is not to say that all women wear shoes their feet don't like for twenty years, but many do, and their feet suffer. The most common problem is that the big toe is forced to deviate towards the middle of the foot, and the joint between the big toe and the foot develops a bunion. At 70, ageing itself does not cause foot problems; a history of the wrong shoes is the cause of problems.

Other problems affect the skin of the foot, principally narrowing of the arteries, both large and small, as a result of disease, for example, in people who have heart disease or diabetes or both.

WHAT YOU CAN DO

By the age of 70 most of us appreciate that our feet are of vital importance and that there are things that we can do to look after them:

- lose weight if you are carrying unnecessary poundage (see page 80)

111

- strengthen the muscles of your lower limbs; strong calf muscles support the arch of the foot because the tendons of the deep calf muscles act like a bowstring to maintain the arch of the foot. See the exercise ideas on pages 45–6

- buy good shoes that allow your feet to be as natural as possible; it is essential to avoid shoes that pinch.

- wash your feet every day, dry them thoroughly, and massage in an oil-based or aqueous cream

- go to see a podiatrist regularly. This is one bit of healthcare many people have to pay for, but it is very good value. You could try to find an NHS podiatrist, but the service is limited and usually concentrates on people at high risk, for example, because of diabetes. Usually weight loss and good foot care can reduce foot problems. Orthotics, devices to fit in your shoe to improve fit and reduce pain, are less important, but may have a part to play.

EARLY WARNING SIGNS

As always, acute pain should not be ignored and the same holds true for ulcers on the skin, particularly for people with diabetes.

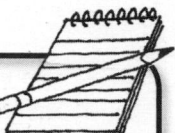

Resolution for better foot maintenance

Write down and stick to a resolution along these lines.

I will:

- not increase my weight from today and, if necessary, will decrease it by keeping to my dietary and stamina resolutions

- do daily exercises to strengthen my leg and foot muscles (see page 47)

- massage aqueous cream into the skin of my feet daily after washing

- *not* cut my toenails myself if I have diabetes. This condition can cause nerve damage and circulation problems which makes cuts and sores hard to heal.

12. Sexual health maintenance

THE EFFECTS OF AGEING

No Sex Please, We're British is the title of a highly successful comedy, and 'no sex please, we're 70' would be just as ridiculous. Physical changes do take place that can reduce both the motivation and the physical ability for sex. Some of these are due to the ageing process, most notably the menopause in women.

In particular the loss of natural lubrication can make sex more difficult and painful but there are steps that can be taken. Firstly, be careful not to let soap or shower gel in the vagina because they can make the dryness worse, wash only with warm water. Secondly, use one of the lubricants that are widely available without prescription. Hormone Replacement Therapy (HRT) can help some people but it carries a risk, so try the simple steps first and then discuss this option with your GP. Book an appointment with a woman partner in the practice if you find it difficult to discuss such things with the male doctor you might usually see.

The existence of an analogous 'male menopause' is not accepted by most scientists. It is true that testosterone levels drop, but the promotion of a syndrome called LowT (low testosterone), which you may have heard of from the manufacturers of testosterone products, is not based on scientific evidence. Advertisements for medication to treat LowT often picture men who are younger than 70 and whose problems are probably either due to diseases, such as Type 2 diabetes, or to drugs, such as those used for heart disease or for psychological reasons rather than the result of reduced hormone levels.

There is a gradual decline in testosterone levels as a result of ageing – about one per cent per year, as is the case with many aspects of ageing. In men, this starts from about 30. There is no sudden drop in the level of the hormones, as there is with female hormones after the onset of the menopause. Despite the facts, the 'manopause' is now a multi-billion-dollar industry in the US. Many men, finding they are gaining weight, are tired and losing interest in sex, have had a blood test which shows a low level of testosterone, which leads, as night follows day, to either a prescription for testosterone or, increasingly, the purchase of testosterone from the web. There is a continuous range of blood testosterone levels just as there is a continuous range of blood pressures or indeed of heights. And just as there is no clear cut-off point between 'low height' and 'high height', or 'low blood pressure' and 'high blood pressure', there appears to be no definite cut-off point between 'low testosterone' and 'normal testosterone'. For some men, Viagra, which is not a form of testosterone, has a contribution to make, but the problem is more often psychological than chemical.

Disease too can reduce both motivation and physical ability, but people aged over 70 are not excluded from a sex life by any rule of nature. The effects of the menopause are partly psychological, but even more important is the effect of the change in hormones on natural lubrication. This can now be countered with easily available lubricants in every pharmacist or online. It is also important to remember that sex is not the be all and end all, and, as Virginia Ironside emphasises in her perceptive and amusing book *The Virginia Monologues: Why Growing Old is Great*, for some people 'the lessening of the sex drive is a bonus'.

WHAT YOU CAN DO

It is hard to distinguish between what is taking place as a result of ageing and what is taking place as a result of the negative stereotyping of people aged 70. These negative views affect some people more than others. You just need to deal with them by reminding yourself that you should not be embarrassed about seeking the advice of a doctor on sexual matters. If you feel there is a problem, consult your doctor, just as you would if you developed difficulties with climbing stairs or passing urine – treat the problem as a physical problem.

EARLY WARNING SIGNS

Regard loss of interest in sex, or difficulty with sex, not as an effect of ageing or a sign of 'growing old', but as a symptom. Ask the advice of your GP in the first instance. For women, if you experience any bleeding after sex, see your GP to exclude any possibility of an illness that needs urgent treatment.

Resolution for better sexual health maintenance

Write down and stick to a resolution along these lines:

- if sexual activity is perceived by me or my partner as a problem, I will seek professional help.

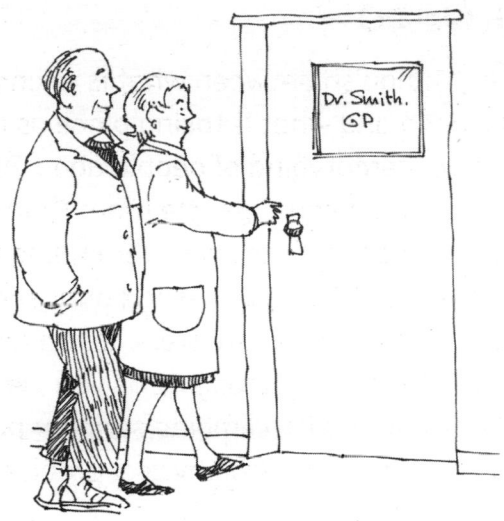

13. Waterworks maintenance

For obvious reasons the maintenance programme for this system differs for men and women.

THE EFFECTS OF AGEING ON WOMEN

The principal reason why some women in their seventies have difficulty passing urine is not because of ageing but because of the birth (or births) of children some forty or fifty years ago. The impact of the head of the foetus on the pelvic floor can have a devastating effect on the muscles of the lower pelvic area. As a result of this, the muscles under the bladder become stretched and weakened. These muscles should hold the urine in the bladder until it is full and then, when the bladder contracts, the urine is pushed through a space in the sheet of muscle and expelled until the bladder is empty. If the muscles have been damaged, the muscles of the pelvic floor do not form a firm barrier under the bladder. The opening of the bladder gapes and some urine can drip into the urethra, the passage to the outside. This creates the sensation of urgency – 'I need to go now' – and, if there is not a toilet nearby, incontinence. Usually this is incontinence of urine, but faecal incontinence can also occur (fortunately this is rarer).

Many women find this very distressing, and even if incontinence does not occur, the feeling of urgency and the possibility that incontinence might occur has a major impact on their quality of life.

THE EFFECTS OF AGEING ON MEN

For men, the villain of the piece is the prostate gland. This gland sits at the junction between the bladder and the urethra, and in most men the gland will grow bigger as you grow older. The reasons for this are not fully understood, but the phenomenon is so common that it can be regarded as an effect of the ageing process. In some men, the enlarged gland interferes with the junction between the bladder and the urethra. As a consequence, urine passes into the urethra even though the bladder is not full and the result is the feeling of urgency and, if they cannot reach a toilet in time, incontinence. Even if incontinence is uncommon, the effects of what is now commonly called LUTS (lower urinary tract symptoms) can affect the quality of life significantly. The symptoms of LUTS include:

- needing to urinate often, both day and night

- difficulty in starting to pass urine

- dribbling at the end of the stream

- a sensation that the bladder is not empty after you think you have finished.

WHAT WOMEN CAN DO

There are now drugs which reduce the feeling of urgency. Sometimes a surgical operation is required and is effective, particularly if there is also a prolapse. However, there is also good evidence that the muscles can be retrained, and although this is most effective immediately after the injury has occurred (that is, in the years following childbirth), it is still worth trying at the age of 70.

Training and retraining the bladder and pelvic floor

- keep a diary of the times you urinate or leak urine for two days

- calculate how many hours you wait between visits to the bathroom during the day

- set your starting interval for training at 15 minutes longer than your typical interval between needing to urinate. So, if you usually make it to one hour before you need to urinate, make your starting interval one hour and fifteen minutes

- on the day you start your training, empty your bladder first thing in the morning and don't go again until you reach your target time interval. If the time arrives before you feel the urge, go anyway. If the urge hits first, remind yourself that your bladder isn't really full, and use whatever techniques you can to delay going

- if you feel the need to go but the interval has not elapsed, try pelvic floor exercises (see opposite), or simply try to wait another five minutes before walking slowly to the bathroom

- increase your interval – once you are successful with your initial interval, increase it by fifteen minutes.

The muscles of the pelvic floor are greatly stretched during childbirth and nowadays it is recognised that women need to be encouraged to regain strength in those muscles in the months after childbirth, but this notion is relatively recent. However, people can regain strength even at 70. Here are the key points of the Kegel exercises, so called because they were developed in the late 1940s by an American gynaecologist, Dr Arnold Kegel:

- identify pelvic floor muscles, by stopping urination in midstream. If you succeed, you can feel the right muscles

- when you've identified the pelvic floor muscles, empty your bladder and lie on your back. Tighten your pelvic floor muscles, hold the contraction for five seconds, and then relax for five seconds. Try five times in a row

- work up to keeping the muscles contracted for 10 seconds at a time, relaxing for ten seconds between contractions

- breathe freely during the exercises

- aim for at least three sets of ten repetitions a day.

Consult your GP if these exercises do not make things better.

WHAT MEN CAN DO

There are fewer things that men can do to deal with the problem of urgency. However, it is sensible to try the bladder retraining technique in the box on pages 119–20. Also, simply use common sense; for example, drink less after 6 p.m.

There are also drugs that can be prescribed for the different symptoms and, in the end, there is prostate surgery, which is getting better and safer. However, prostate surgery carries risks, so you need to be sure, first, that the problem is really bothering you and, second, you have tried everything possible before surgery. Your doctor can advise about these issues.

EARLY WARNING SIGNS

Lower urinary tract symptoms are themselves early warning signs of prostate trouble if you are a man and pelvic floor problems if you are a woman, and you should seek help if the self help measures we recommend are unsuccessful. The only serious sign of other disease is the sudden appearance of blood in the urine; that should be discussed with your GP. The acute or sudden onset of incontinence should also be referred to your doctor.

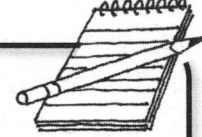

Resolution for better waterworks maintenance

Write down and stick to a resolution along these lines.

I will:

- keep as fit as possible

- follow a routine of bladder training at least once a day if I have developed any difficulty

- do my pelvic floor exercises every day.

14. Tooth and gum maintenance

THE EFFECTS OF AGEING

Not much change occurs after your adult teeth have arrived. The teeth do not produce new cells, but nor are they affected much by the process of ageing because there is little metabolism or cell division taking place. It is amazing that we still have teeth at the age of 70; it is like having a china dinner service for sixty years. And the teeth, like a dinner service, come in for some pretty rough handling.

Many of us in our seventies remember the day when sugar rationing ended and, for many of us, the next ten years were spent with sugar in our mouths, usually in the form of sweets like gobstoppers that lasted as long as possible. Even without these, teeth have a tough time. Even the most careful person may bite on something very hard, and many of us eat between meals, snack on biscuits or even eat apples without thinking about the effect on our teeth.

Furthermore, our teeth have to spend their life in one of the unhealthiest places in the body – the mouth. Even the best kept mouth is full of bacteria, and these bacteria attack the vulnerable border zone between the teeth and the gums. This leads to the formation of what is called plaque at this junction, which can lead to inflammation of the gums – gingivitis. This, in turn, leads to shrinkage of the gums, which can mean that even if our teeth are undamaged, they are no longer strongly anchored. In our seventies, more teeth are lost through

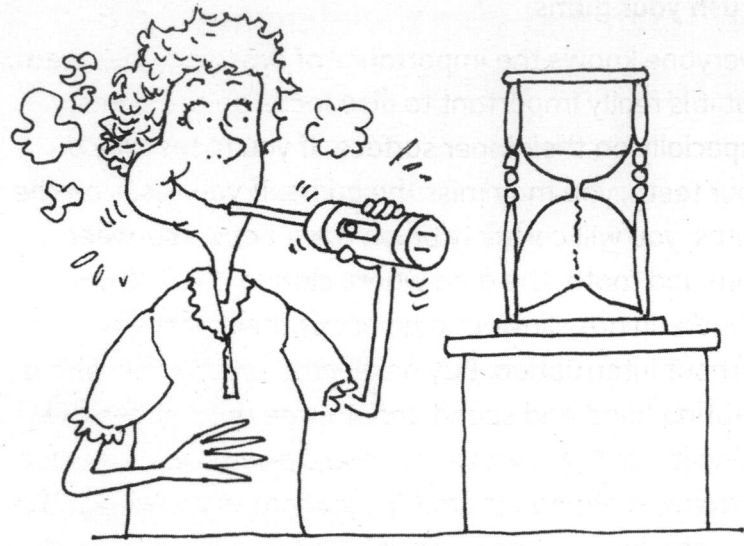

gum disease than through disease affecting the teeth directly. Therefore, the teeth that have survived need obsessional care, as do the gums. Assess how much time you spend looking after your teeth and gums at present. For most people the time spent needs to be increased by three to five times. It is not unreasonable to spend up to ten minutes a day on the little devils.

WHAT YOU CAN DO

There are four things to focus on:

- brush your gums
- minimise sugar and acid
- get the benefits of fluoride
- visit your dental hygenist regularly.

Brush your gums

Everyone knows the importance of brushing your teeth, but it is really important to also focus on the gums, especially on their inner surface. If you focus only on your teeth, you may miss the gums. If you focus on the gums, you will certainly brush the junction between gum and tooth, the area where plaque is laid down if bacteria are allowed to go about their business without interruption. Buy an electric toothbrush with a rotating head and spend about three or four minutes using it night and morning – more often if you can, but certainly night and morning if you are still working. This is necessary but not sufficient. You also need to brush between the teeth with little single-pronged brushes, which are available from chemists and supermarkets.

- if you can't get through, use dental floss and then return to the attack

- if you see blood, keep going – in fact, redouble your efforts, however, if bleeding persists see your dentist or doctor.

Even if you have a plate replacing some of your teeth, love those that are remaining like ewe lambs.

Love your gums, but not with tender love; they like it rough! Only the rough treatment displaces food particles and the bacteria that flourish upon them.

Minimise sugar and acid

- avoid sugar, not just the total amount but the frequency of use – this is important

- avoid acid, for example, in fruit juice or fizzy drinks, and if you do eat acidic food, such as an apple, neutralise the effects of the acid with alkali such as a piece of cheese.

Get the benefits of fluoride

- use fluoride toothpaste

- use fluoride mouthwash at least once a day, at different times from the brushing

- visit your dental hygenist at least twice a year.

EARLY WARNING SIGNS

One important early warning of trouble is your nearest and dearest complaining about the noise you make grinding your teeth when asleep! Grinding can crack fillings and even shatter teeth, so see a dentist to get what is called a guard or splint.

Remember to consult a dentist or your GP if you have a mouth ulcer that does not heal in three weeks.

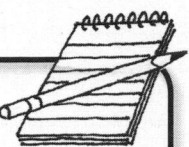

Resolution for better tooth and gum health

Write down and stick to a resolution along these lines.

Every day I will:

- brush my teeth and gums with an electric toothbrush twice a day for at least four minutes each time

- use a fluoride mouthwash once a day

- clean between my teeth with an interdental brush, or floss if I cannot get a brush through, at least once a day.

15. Skin maintenance

The colour of your hair is easy to deal with, ageing skin is more of a challenge!

THE EFFECTS OF AGEING

Ageing skin has:

- fewer elastic fibres

- fewer sweat glands

- fewer sebaceous glands producing natural oil.

However, the resulting wrinkles and blemishes are principally due to exposure to the elements, particularly sunshine. Look at the skin on the inside of your upper arm, and you will see smooth and young-looking skin.

WHAT YOU CAN DO

There are two essential steps you can take:

- protect yourself from the sun

- apply moisturising cream, preferably oil-based.

It is still vitally important at the age of 70 to protect your skin from the harmful effects of the sun and the

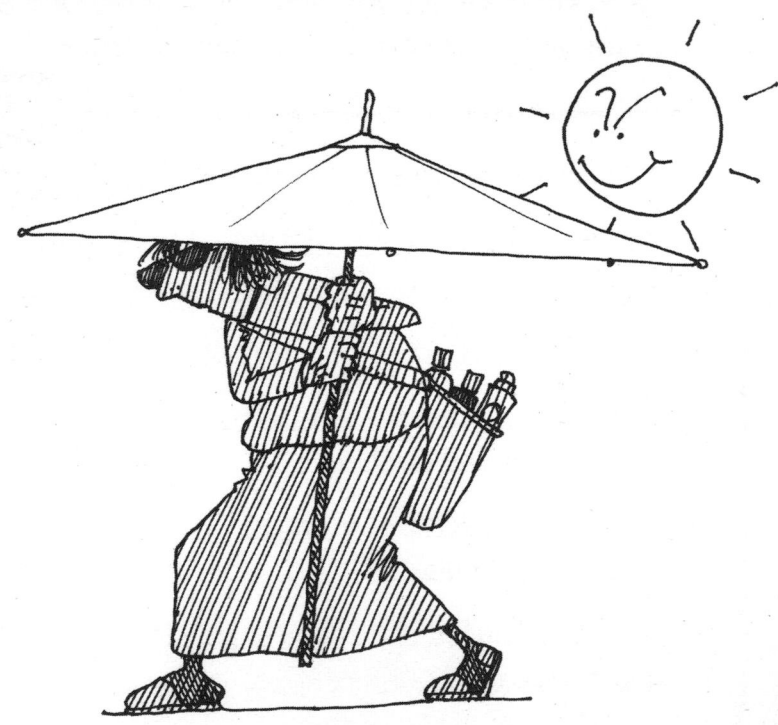

risk of skin cancer. It is true there is a beneficial effect from vitamin D formation from sunlight, but you can also take a tablet of 15–20mg a day.

- always use sun-screen, at least a factor 20

- keep covered up

- buy a big tub of moisturiser, preferably oil rather than water based, and massage it all over your skin regularly – if possible once a day, but at least once a week. Concentrate particularly on those areas which have been exposed to the sun. It does not matter which oil is the base, and there is no need to pay a lot of money. The best value is usually a low-cost, paraffin-based cream.

Resolution for better skin maintenance

Write down and stick to a resolution along these lines.

I will:

- protect my skin from the sun by wearing sun-screen and clothing

- use an oil-based cream all over your body at least once a week

- use an oil-based cream on exposed skin at least once a day.

EARLY WARNING SIGNS

There are two important early warning signs of skin cancer:

- an ulcer, particularly on your face or lip, that fails to heal after a month

- a mole that changes size or shape, or starts to bleed.

Always consult your doctor about these problems.

16. Vision maintenance

Vision and hearing are of vital importance, not just for independence, but also for mental wellbeing.

THE EFFECTS OF AGEING

Vision changes as a result of ageing. The lens of the eye becomes less elastic, and almost everyone needs spectacles for reading when they can no longer hold the book far enough away to compensate for the lack of elasticity (almost everyone, but not everyone; Menahem Pressler at the age of 90 could still read the blizzard of notes in Mozart piano concerto scores without glasses or contact lenses).

Ageing also contributes to three of the four major eye diseases in old age: glaucoma (a build up of pressure in the eye), cataract (development of a cloudy patch across the lens) and macular degeneration (a gradual loss of central, but not peripheral, vision) are all found more commonly in the older age groups (the fourth major eye disease is a complication of diabetes). These conditions are common, but not universal, so either there is some additional factor that determines which of us will develop the disease or some genetic factor which either increases or decreases the risk. Fortunately, there are now effective treatments for these diseases.

WHAT YOU CAN DO

It is sensible to have an eye test every two years. For some people who suffer only from difficulty with reading, it is possible to buy reading spectacles in a shop, but a professional eye examination can detect other diseases. It is important to appreciate that in eye care, as in any other branch of healthcare, diagnosis does not necessarily indicate a need for treatment, and just because an optometrist identifies early cataract or raised intraocular pressure (a sign that serious glaucoma might develop), this does not mean you need treatment immediately, or even ever.

EARLY WARNING SIGNS

If you notice any gradual change in your vision (such as difficulty reading number plates of cars while driving), make an appointment to get your eyes tested. Any sudden loss of vision, complete or even partial, is an emergency and requires a visit to the nearest hospital (a specialist eye hospital, if possible, or otherwise a general A&E department).

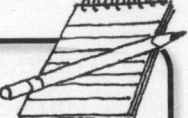

Resolution for better vision maintenance

Write down and stick to a resolution along these lines:

- I will have my eyes examined every two years (write down the date of your last examination on the resolution so you know when to book the next one).

17. Hearing maintenance

Loss of hearing is regarded with less sympathy than loss of sight, but age-related hearing loss (ARHL) can be just as disabling as visual impairment.

THE EFFECTS OF AGEING

From childhood onwards, hearing loss occurs, initially for high-pitched sounds, but in later life all pitches may be affected. Hearing is carried out by very delicate organs in the middle and inner ear, and the changes that take place in the inner ear, in what is called the organ of Corti, are responsible for most of the cases of ARHL. Unlike impairment in the function of the lungs or heart, there is little evidence that ARHL is caused by disease except for the small number of people with industrial deafness. It is an effect of ageing that occurs more quickly in some people than in others, for reasons that are probably genetic. The psychological and physical complications that follow the development of ARHL can be significant, so treat loss of hearing as a serious problem.

Hearing loss may be accompanied by tinnitus – annoying sounds that may occur as a result of changes in the nervous system – or it can occur alone. The first sign is often that we can't hear others speaking when there is background noise, at a party for example, but if the problem comes on gradually we may be unaware. It is other people around us who will notice changes, such as playing the TV or radio at high volume, or failing to hear the doorbell.

WHAT YOU CAN DO

There is no screening programme for hearing loss in older people, although many people argue that there should be. Detection and treatment therefore depend on you taking action of your own accord, unless you are prompted to do so by someone else who has noticed your difficulty hearing things.

Anyone can make an appointment with their GP, but he or she will probably simply refer you to the audiology service of the local hospital, or to an approved provider of NHS hearing aids such as Specsavers. The charity Action on Hearing Loss, formerly the Royal National Institute for Deaf People, runs an excellent assessment service online at www.actiononhearingloss.org.uk that includes a hearing test and advice on how to find an audiology service. It is important that you are clear about the service being offered because hearing aids (or hearing instruments as they are sometimes called) dispensed by an audiologist on the high street may not be funded by the NHS.

For some people, the principal problem is wax, but you should not put anything smaller than your finger in your ear; don't go poking about with matchsticks or cotton buds, go to someone who is trained to deal with earwax (consult your doctor in the first instance).

EARLY WARNING SIGNS

Difficulty in hearing children or women talking is often the earliest sign of ARHL because they speak at a higher pitch. The cause may simply be wax, but go and see your GP for advice.

Resolution for better hearing maintenance

Write down and stick to a resolution along these lines:

- I will seek help when someone says 'You have the television awfully loud' or some such comment, which could indicate hearing loss, or if I become aware of having difficulty hearing things.

4

CHOOSING AND USING HEALTHCARE WISELY

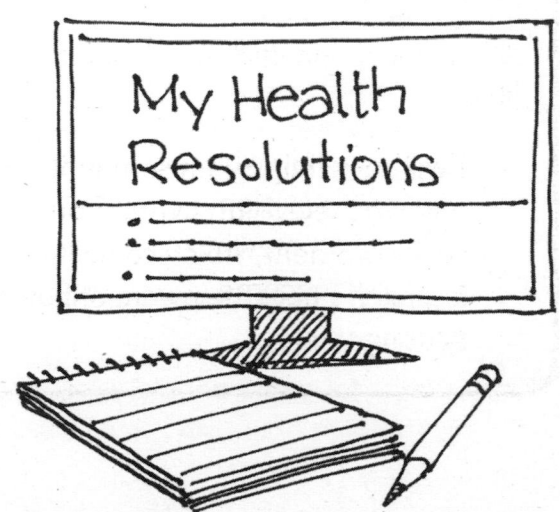

Power to the People

The more we know about our health, the more power we have. It is astonishing how many tests and treatments are now available to the medical profession. The sad fact is that many of us are receiving too much medical intervention – treatments that are of little benefit, and may, in fact, be doing us harm.

Too much medicine

It comes as a surprise to many people that doctors are cautious users of health services, despite benefiting from several advantages not available to the wider population:

- doctors know about the fantastic progress that has been made in medical care in the last fifty years

- they receive the best information about the benefits of new treatments.

- they could get referred to the doctor considered to be the best for a particular operation or treatment by the medical profession.

The reasons for their caution are many, but they include:

- knowing that a medical intervention – a test, an operation or a drug – always has harmful side effects for some people, even when carried out by the best doctor in the country.

- knowing that there is usually more scientific evidence available about the benefit of a new treatment than the amount of evidence about its risks and limitations. Trials of a new treatment that have produced a positive result and show a benefit are more likely to be published than reports of trials of the same drug that did not have a positive result.

Doctors also know that harm can occur even in the best services.

- laboratory, screening, or radiological investigations often produce what are called false positive results, suggesting that disease is present when it is not. This leads to follow-up tests and treatments that can be risky and harmful. CT scanning itself raises the risk of cancer because of radiation

- some surgical operations are necessary for every patient: doctors would agree that an operation for someone with bowel cancer is essential. Other operations are only necessary for some people with a condition such as a cataract or arthritis of the knee. Both the doctor and the patient have to decide whether the operation is appropriate for that individual. The reason for considering the appropriateness of the treatment for the individual is that even very good interventions leave a small proportion of patients with some adverse effect. The better the surgeon and operating team, the lower the proportion of people who have such an effect, but all operations can do harm as well as good, and if the operation was not essential in the first place then the patient has to live with the regret of having made the wrong choice

- all drugs can have harmful side-effects, spelled out in great detail in very small print in a leaflet within the box in which the drugs are dispensed, but this only becomes clear after the prescription has been collected from the pharmacist.

Modern medicine has amazing tests and treatments – magnetic resonance imaging (MRI, which is replacing X-rays), transplants, hip replacements and chemotherapy, to give but a few examples – but there is growing concern among the medical profession itself about over-diagnosis and over-treatment.

The *British Medical Journal* is playing a leading part in a campaign called Too Much Medicine, which claims 'to highlight the threat to human health posed by over-diagnosis and the waste of resources on unnecessary care ... for a wide range of conditions such as prostate and thyroid cancers, asthma and chronic kidney disease.' The problem is much greater in some other countries than in the UK, notably in the United States, where an excellent book by Nortin M. Hadler was published in 2011 called *Rethinking Aging: Growing Old and Living Well in an Overtreated Society.*

Not enough medicine

It is also important to emphasise that there is sometimes an underuse of medical treatment because of ageism. Attitudes are changing, especially as it is now recognised that many of the health problems older people experience are not caused by the ageing process. However, far too often, people are told 'it's your age' or even asked 'what else can you expect at your age?' Old age is *not* a diagnosis. The doctor who says such things is ageist and prejudiced if he assumes that all the patient's problems are caused by the ageing process. Medical ageism is now recognised as a problem that the medical profession has to tackle. Older patients should never be referred to as 'bed-blockers' or 'crumblies'. You should be addressed by your proper name rather than 'pet' or 'lovey', or some other familiar term that may be well intentioned but which would never be used with a patient who was a 40-year-old accountant or a 50-year-old architect.

I would encourage you to always challenge your doctor if you feel in any way dissatisfied or unclear about what you are being told. That said, I understand that challenging people in positions of authority can be difficult to do. You may find it easier to express your concerns indirectly, for example, by saying, 'I was reading about this problem on NHS Choices, you know the patients' website ...' or even 'my daughter told me to ask you about ...'

Remember – ageing is not a disease, and old age is not a diagnosis.

Getting the right care for you

In your seventies you need to maximise the benefits you get from modern medicine while minimising the harms. Set out below are a few methods for achieving this.

- be clear about what matters most to you

- ask for clear, high-quality information on the risks and benefits of relevant tests and treatments

- do your own research

- take sufficient time to reflect on which option is best for you.

BE CLEAR ABOUT WHAT MATTERS MOST TO YOU

Mrs Johnson thanked the doctor, and left the consulting room to look for some other solution to what mattered most to her – problems with gardening. There was no doubt that Mrs Johnson had arthritis of the knee joint, but the solution for her was not a knee replacement, which might well have resulted in her being unable to kneel at all. As her problem was primarily her difficulty with gardening, a raised flower bed might be the solution, or long-handled garden tools.

Before going to see your GP or, even more importantly, a specialist who does not know you in the way that your GP does, think and then write down your thoughts and concerns.

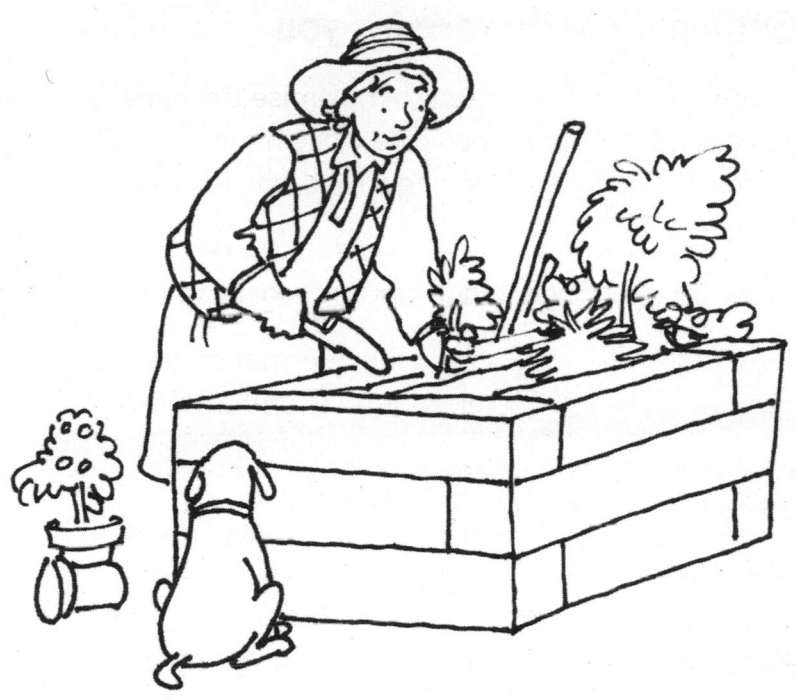

For example, if you are feeling tired but are really worried that you may have developed cancer, the box would look like this.

What is really bothering me most?	I am worried that I might have cancer because I seem more tired
What do I hope the health service can do about it?	Exclude the possibility that the cause of my tiredness is cancer (although nothing is ever 100 per cent certain in medicine)

ASK FOR CLEAR, HIGH-QUALITY INFORMATION

For a variety of reasons, the information given to patients is sometimes overly optimistic regarding the risks and limitations of treatment. This is changing, but over-optimism is a very deep-seated tendency. Perhaps the main obstacle is the use of percentages. We know that if people are told that a treatment will reduce the risk of a disease by 50 per cent, they make different decisions than if they are told that the risk will be reduced from 1 in 2,000 to 1 in 3,000. You need absolute numbers, so here are two questions for your doctor:

- if 100 people have this test or treatment, how many of them will have a good result?

- if 100 people have this test or treatment, how many of them will suffer some harmful consequence?

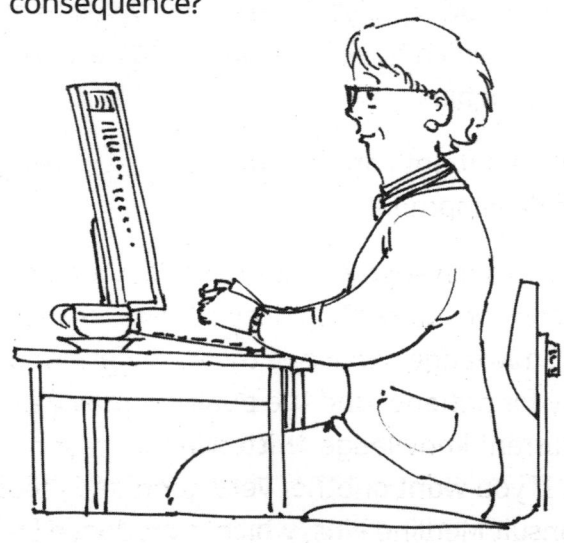

DO YOUR OWN RESEARCH

The Internet is wonderful, but it also creates problems. I put 'knee replacement' into Google in June 2014 and got 24,400,000 results. The top results are usually a reflection of how much the websites paid to achieve that ranking rather than the quality or suitability of the website. How do you find information that you are sure you can rely on?

If you are considering any kind of treatment, the best sources of information:

- are unconnected to any related commercial interest

- use standardised methods to assess the strength of the evidence on which their information is based

- use methods to display risks and benefits of the options which have been shown by research to minimise bias

- involve patients and the public in their design and development.

There are two such sources that I can recommend. First, you can consult NHS Choices at www.nhs.uk – this is the knowledge service of the NHS, designed specifically for patients and the public. It provides the best current knowledge written in non-technical language. If you want another very good and reliable source, consult Medline Plus, which is produced by the world's greatest medical library, the National Library of Medicine in Washington DC, at www.nlm.nih.gov/medlineplus.

TAKE SUFFICIENT TIME TO REFLECT

So how do you make a decision about the right treatment for you?

- look at the evidence about the risks and benefits as shown in studies of patients with the same condition

- consider the specific nature of your own particular condition – you may have more than one disease or other factors to take into account

- think about what is important to you.

All of these elements need to be weighed up for you to decide the value you place on the benefits and harms associated with any treatment.

'What would you do, doctor?' is a question often asked. This is a difficult question for a doctor because there are in fact two questions:

- what would you do if you were me?

- what would you do, doctor?

The answer that a doctor could give to the first question, if he or she were willing to commit themselves, would depend on many things, principally on his or her knowledge of you and your values. Notably:

- what value you would place on the different outcomes, both good and bad?

- how do you feel about risk-taking?

- how would you feel if you had taken a risk and it had turned out badly?

But what about the answer to the second question? Although doctors are highly trained about medical matters, when they are patients, they use the same three questions as you do. They think about the problems they face, the risks and benefits of the options they face and how they feel about taking risk. It does seem that doctors are more concerned about the risks of treatments. They know that things can go wrong, even in the best of services, and of course they can often remember a particular patient for whom the treatment turned out badly. What doctors are now appreciating is the need to focus on you, the individual, not the disease. In many ways, this is a return to a more old fashioned approach. You need to be clear about what is bothering you most and weigh up the benefits and risks, because all treatment carries a risk, and the decision whether to have a particular treatment does not require a medical degree.

You need to take your time and reflect by yourself, and with family and friends, using the checklist below:

- what is bothering me most?

- is the doctor clear about what is bothering me most?

- will the treatment being offered not just treat the disease but deal with what is bothering me most?

- am I well informed about the probability of benefit and the probability of harm?

Having decided on this, you need to consider a number of other questions:

- am I really sure I want this treatment? (I know this is a repeat but it is always worth revisiting)

- will I blame myself if it does go wrong?

- what have other people like me decided? (Look at two very good websites: www.patientslikeme. com and www.healthtalkonline.co.uk)

- how urgently is the treatment needed?

- where should I have it done?

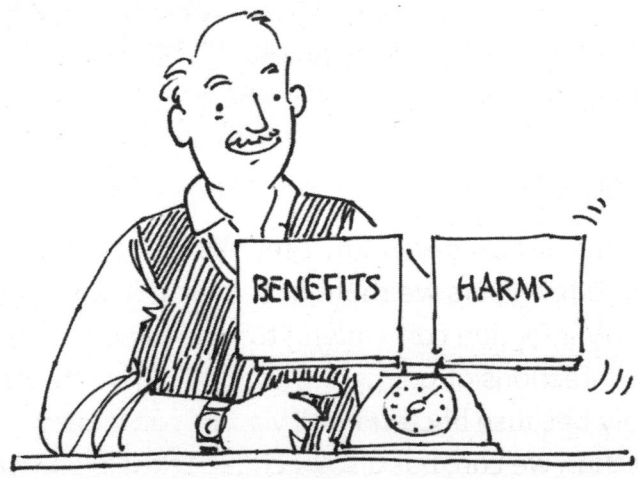

Increasingly, hospitals are publishing the results of treatment services. Look at www.nhs.uk to see if there is any information about the treatment you are considering, and the performance of the hospitals that provide the treatment within a reasonable distance of where you live.

Right care for people aged 70 plus

The previous section emphasised how important it is to personalise decision-making. Health services certainly need clear firm guidelines about how to diagnose and treat disease, but each of us is unique. Our unique clinical condition, the presence or absence of other risk factors, and the presence of any other conditions all need to be taken into account, along with our values. It is, however, possible to make some generalisations – not to state that everyone aged 70 should or must have this test or treatment, but that everyone aged 70 must be given information about certain tests or treatments. It is then up to each of us to decide if that test or treatment is right for us.

VACCINATION

Infectious diseases were the great killers of the past, and for a few years we thought they had gone away. Then HIV infection came along to remind us that we ignore infections at our peril. That peril has increased, not only because bacteria and viruses can evolve faster than we can, but also because of the over-use of antibiotics, which has led to the development of antibiotic resistance. Fortunately, we have effective vaccines against some of the predominant diseases that occur in old age.

There are three diseases that can be prevented by immunisation:

- influenza

- pneumococcal pneumonia

- shingles.

Influenza

For two reasons, influenza for people in their seventies and older influenza is a much more serious condition than for people at the age of 30. First, the effects of ageing reduce our capacity to respond to challenges. The identical challenge, in this case the influenza virus, has a bigger impact the older the person is, so influenza, which may result in three days off work for a 30-year-old, may lead to three days in hospital for a person aged 70 or over. Second (and this is obviously inter-related with the first reason), people over 70 may already have changes in their lungs and heart as a result of lifestyle and environment, and the added burden of influenza can lead to problems in both. One function of the heart is to pump blood through the lungs to collect oxygen. If the lungs become infected and inflamed, the heart has more work to do, and this can precipitate heart failure. For these reasons, influenza immunisation should be seriously considered by everyone aged over 70.

Pneumococcal pneumonia

Staphylococcus pneumoniae is a bacterium that causes a serious type of pneumonia. Fortunately, a safe and effective vaccine now exists – the pneumococcal polysaccharide vaccine (PPV). Everyone aged 65 should have been offered this vaccine at some stage, because it gives lifetime protection to people who have no other health problems. People who have long-term conditions of the heart, lungs or kidneys, or who have diabetes (and are therefore at higher risk of complications), should have it every five years.

Shingles

Shingles is a very nasty affliction. It flares up when some change in your body leads to a reactivation of the chickenpox virus which has lain dormant or been sleeping inside your nervous system. The trigger factor is not clearly understood, but there is now a vaccine that is being offered to people aged 70 and over – the group at highest risk.

REDUCING RISKS

'Nothing is certain except death and taxes' is the great phrase first used by Daniel Defoe, author of *Robinson Crusoe* (although the Americans give credit for the saying to Benjamin Franklin). Disease develops more commonly as age increases, but it is not inevitable. The best way to think is that a person at 70 is certainly at increased risk of disease, but many of these diseases can be prevented, postponed or made less severe. These include:

- heart disease – heart attacks and heart failure

- stroke

- the type of dementia called vascular dementia, due to disease of the blood vessels, and atrial fibrillation, a disorder of the heart which causes the heart to beat irregularly. This allows little clots to form in the heart, which can then break off and be carried in the bloodstream to the brain

- kidney failure and other complications of Type 2 Diabetes

- severe joint disease necessitating joint replacement

- cancer

- depression.

Some risk factors are common to more than one disease. The risks can be reduced by the following actions:

- stopping smoking

- improving your diet

- losing weight

- becoming more active and fitter
- using your skills and resources to help others less fortunate than you are.

Many of these actions can be carried out by you, using the advice and techniques offered throughout this book, but balance this with the need to be aware of any risk factors that may require further investigation by a doctor.

PREVENTIVE SERVICES

Before undertaking any exercise programme, it is a good idea to ask your doctor for a health check. There is no need to spend money on privately advertised screening tests, or whole-body scans, as there is strong evidence that they do more harm than good. In addition, the NHS can provide preventive services for people aged 70 and over, in particular for the following:

- detection and treatment of high blood pressure
- detection and treatment of an irregular heartbeat (atrial fibrillation)
- prevention and management of Type 2 diabetes
- prompt investigation of acute chest pain to treat heart attacks effectively
- screening tests for breast cancer for women, for abdominal aortic aneurysm for men (see page 94), and for bowel cancer for both

- investigation, treatment and follow-up for women who have had one fracture, to prevent a second fragility fracture

- identification of depression, and effective treatment and support to improve wellbeing and prevent suicide.

What is needed, then, is a balanced approach. We need to be offered high-value treatment, but it is essential also to avoid over-diagnosis, over-treatment and the medicalisation of life.

LIVING HEALTHILY WITH A CHRONIC CONDITION

Many people will develop a disease in their seventies, some more than one. But what is a disease? Some are clear-cut. Tuberculosis is a disease; so too is a myocardial infarction (a heart attack). But not all diseases are so obvious.

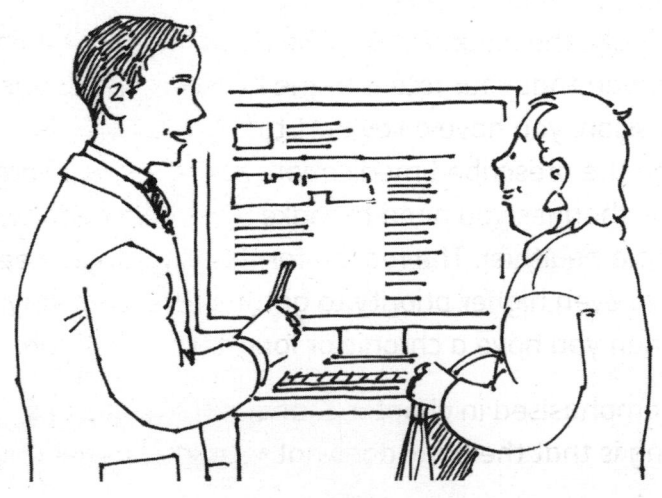

Take high blood pressure, for example. All of us have a blood pressure that is high enough to drive the arterial blood to where it is needed; without it we would be dead. But in some people, the level of pressure becomes so high that it is judged sensible to prescribe medication to reduce it, in order to lower the risk of heart disease and stroke. Giving this condition the name 'high blood pressure' makes it simpler for someone to say 'I have high blood pressure' rather than: 'Well, my doctor and I agreed that my level of blood pressure is such that the reduction in risk of having a stroke justifies the possible side-effects of taking medication every day to reduce my average blood pressure.' High blood pressure is a condition, rather than a disease. So too is Type 2 diabetes, and so are a number of other 'conditions'. The onset of a condition – or the diagnosis of a disease – is not the end.

Even the diagnosis of a disease like cancer is not the end; it is, in fact, the beginning of a new journey. Obviously, the diagnosis may be depressing, but it does not mean that your fate is in the hands of the medical profession: you have a key part to play, not only in taking the prescribed medication, but in taking charge of the changes you need to make to remain healthy, or become healthier. The reason for this is that you need to give even higher priority to getting fitter and staying fit when you have a chronic or long-term condition.

As I emphasised in chapter 1, one of the effects of ageing is that the body does not respond so well to the challenge of inactivity, so that you lose fitness more easily the older you get. When you develop a chronic condition, two other factors come into play:

- first, the effects of the disease itself, joint pain or breathlessness for example, may make movement and activity more difficult

- second, you have to resist the pressures of other people who, with the best of intentions, want to do things for you when, in fact, it would be better for you to do them yourself.

For these reasons, not only does the best possible rate of decline accelerate due to the disease process, but there may be an even faster decline in the actual rate of decline due to social pressures to 'take things easier'.

For this reason, fitness – both physical and psychological – becomes even more important for those of us with one or more long-term conditions than for people who do not have them, or who have not yet developed them. For all the common serious conditions that occur in your seventies and eighties, there is now good evidence of the benefits of being more active. These are the same activities that reduce the risk of disease in the first place – a healthier, high-fibre diet, and increased activity we've talked about in earlier chapters.

These health-promoting behaviours are equally important for conditions that we cannot at present prevent, such as Parkinson's disease, and it is essential to emphasise their importance after the diagnosis has been made, as well as prescribing drug treatment. If you have been diagnosed with cancer, you may need some combination of surgery, chemotherapy and radiotherapy, but you should also try to remain active, improve your diet and learn techniques such as mindfulness (see page 176).

Unless you are lucky enough to be referred to a physiotherapist or exercise therapist, you may have to do this yourself by following the guidance in chapter 2. You can discuss this with your doctor to make sure that trying to get fitter will not cause you any harm. Also, patient charities such as Macmillan Cancer Support and the British Heart Foundation are right up to speed with facts and figures, and are playing a leading part in promoting the health of people with chronic disease. Macmillan Cancer Support finances health walks, organised by the Ramblers, not only for people with cancer but for all those who have long-term conditions (see www.walkingforhealth.org.uk).

Use medicines wisely

Modern medicine has been transformed by the development of new drugs, as well as by advances in diagnostics and surgery, but medicine, like all other treatments, can do harm from their side effects. Of course, side effects only affect a proportion of people taking a particular drug, and many are relatively minor, such as a skin rash. The leaflets provided by the drug companies contain a large amount of information, often in very small print, but it is difficult to find information about the possible side effect of taking a combination of two or more drugs. For this type of information, and for all questions relating to the use of a drug, its effects and side effects, the best source of information is your pharmacist.

What about alternative and complementary medicine?

Some doctors are very critical of treatments like homeopathy or Chinese medicine, particularly if they take NHS resources that could otherwise be spent on services such as hip replacements. Their criticism stems from the fact that these treatments are not based on strong evidence of effectiveness, which is normally evidence produced from systematic reviews of a type of research called randomised controlled trials. In response, the providers of complementary and alternative medicines argue that they would be willing to do more research, but that there is no equivalent of the pharmaceutical industry, which funds so much of the research on new drugs.

So what can be said if you are considering such a treatment? First, we can say that many people have benefited from alternative and complementary treatments. Second, there is little evidence that these treatments do harm, provided that you do not stop taking an orthodox treatment of proven effectiveness.

Ensuring the right care at the end of life

As one reaches 70, losing friends and relatives makes the inevitability of death for us all creep up the agenda. At least one parent or other elderly relative of people in their sixties and seventies may still be living, and responsibility for their care often rests with their children. Sharing experiences of loss can be comforting, and enables people to talk more easily and openly about what has long been for many a taboo subject. It can also be a great help to the recently bereaved to share their experience of events *prior* to death, such as the difficulties in obtaining the right type of care at home, or finding a good caring environment elsewhere, or whether the last days of a person's death were marred by perhaps unnecessary medical interventions. In the back of our minds it raises the question of how we ourselves would wish to be cared for at the end of our life, and what preparations we should make to ensure what is called a 'good death'. But what is a 'good death'?

Bill Shankly, the famous manager of Liverpool Football Club, said that his ambition was to 'die healthy'. Like many people, his concern was to be active and independent, and have a good life, until near the end. The core message of this book is that by taking action, it is possible to remain active and independent for longer, not necessarily to extend life, but to postpone the onset of disability and dependence on others, and reduce its duration from years to months, if not weeks.

The concept of 'a good death' concentrates more on the last weeks, days or hours of life, when it is clear that death is near. How this critical time can best be managed is at last becoming a matter for much more open debate and discussion. A sudden death may seem to some to be ideal, but can have its drawbacks, notably the loss of an opportunity not only to say goodbye to those one loves, but also to make it up with people with whom there might have been a disagreement. Professor Ira Byock, an American palliative care specialist, wisely identifies that most people want to have the opportunity before they die to talk about 'the four things that matter most: please forgive me; I forgive you; I love you. Thank you.'

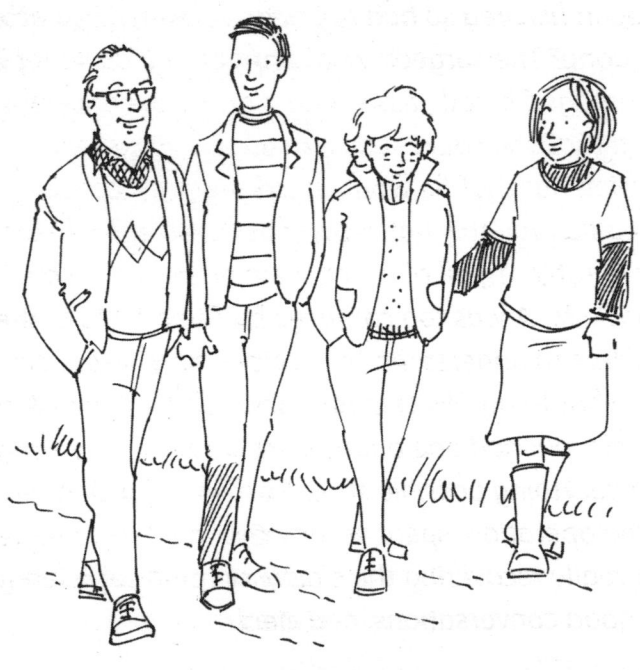

The last days of life can also be spoiled by what is called 'inappropriate' or 'futile' medical care.

Mr A was 76 and healthy. Sure, he had a few medical problems, and lots of prescriptions, but he had a good life with his wife of fifty years. He was secretary of his local community centre, a keen bowler, and an active member of the Allotment Committee. Then one day he collapsed with very severe abdominal pain and was taken to the local hospital where the diagnosis was made of a ruptured abdominal aneurysm. An aortic aneurysm can be treated with a low risk if detected before the aneurysm bursts, and, for this reason, there is a screening programme offered to men aged 65. But Mr A had been above that age when the programme had started in his area so had not been screened. What was to be done? The surgeon was confident he could replace the damaged blood vessel with a graft, the anaesthetist agreed that she could keep him alive through the operation but that he would need days in intensive care and would probably not recover because of his heart and kidney problems, all of which were being aggravated by shock. Mr A was too confused by the effects of the painkillers to understand the options fully. Mrs A did not know what to do. His children, who lived in the USA and Australia, phoned one another and argued very strongly that 'everything possible should be done for Dad', so he had the operation, spent seven days in intensive care, never really recovering the clarity of mind sufficiently to have good conversations, and died.

We hear a great deal about physician assisted suicide, but Mr A's case was one example of a much more common problem – physician-assisted survival. He survived the operation, so the surgeon could classify it as a 'success', but died, as most doctors would have predicted, seven days later. His treatment was all done with the best of intentions, but what would Mr A have wanted? No one knew, so the safest decision was made: to try everything.

Fortunately, the problem of over-diagnosis, and over-treatment is now recognised, particularly in the United States, where authors such as Nortin M. Hadler, have emphasised that the current approach, which sees hospitalisation as the right thing to do for acutely ill elderly people near the end of life, is a policy that is 'more lethal than it is salutary' – in other words more likely to do harm than good. Many people do not want to be admitted to hospital at what may be the end of their life, particularly when there is no guarantee that the treatment will work and a high probability that the treatment and its consequences will make the process of dying worse. What can be done about this?

The first step is to discuss these issues. The subject of death and dying is one which many of us are reluctant to raise, but discussion is essential, particularly with those closest such as a spouse, a child, or other relatives. Obviously religious beliefs will also have a very important part to play, and even people who are not formally religious may have spiritual needs and concerns to be taken into account. Decisions are highly personal and individual, and each of us must approach this in our own way. It seems that more people are now thinking about and discussing issues such as:

- what do I want to happen at the end of life?

- what don't I want to happen?

- who will speak for me and act on my behalf if I cannot do so myself.

There are a number of specific issues that need to be considered, such as:

- do you want to be resuscitated if, for example, you have a cardiac arrest after you have had a major stroke?

- are there specific treatments you do *not* want to have, for example, if you were to develop dementia, would you want to have external cardiac massage and electrical defibrillation if your heart were to suddenly stop, or would you want antibiotic treatment if you developed pneumonia when it might be that pneumonia would be a peaceful way of leaving this world?

- who could make decisions for you if you became incompetent and unable to make decisions that were legally valid about whether or not to have an operation that could not guarantee success and carried some risk, as a result of becoming unconscious, for example?

These decisions overlap and it is sensible to assume that you will need to nominate someone who is authorised to act on your behalf. If you are calm and fully alert, you can discuss options with the medical team caring for you, but it is often the case that at the time when serious decisions have to be made, your ability to make them may be compromised by your condition. Many people are now taking steps to state their views for 'when the time comes', in discussion with their family, realising it is often one's closest relations that have to make these difficult decisions unless the person's views are clear.

Not everyone wishes to make these decisions in advance, however, and this has to be respected. Often, of course, different members of the family may have different views, and this can lead to argument and conflict, which in turn makes a demanding situation even more difficult. A solution that can be chosen is to make an 'advance decision to refuse treatment' (previously known as an 'advance directive'). This decision is made when you have the 'capacity' to make it and can be used later if you are unable to make the decision at the time of the proposed medical treatment. If you wish to refuse life-sustaining or life-saving treatments in circumstances where you might die as a result of this refusal, the treatments you would refuse must all be named in the advance decision, for example that:

- you would not want antibiotics for an infection if you were only expected to live for a few days

- you would not want to be kept alive by being fed and given fluids through a nasal tube or a drip if you were unable to swallow food and drink

- you would not want anyone to try to restart your heart by electric shock or cardiac massage if your heart stopped beating.

You may find it helpful to talk to a doctor or nurse about the kinds of treatments you might be offered in the future, and what it might mean if you choose not to have them.

You must write down:

- your name, date of birth, address and any distinguishing features – in case you are unable to communicate and healthcare professionals need to identify you

- the name, address and phone number of your GP, and whether or not they have a copy of your advance decision to refuse treatment document.

- a statement saying that the document should be used if you ever lack capacity to make decisions

- a statement about which treatments are to be refused, including the words 'I refuse this treatment even if my life is at risk as a result'

- the date

- your signature

- a dated signature of at least one witness

As an indication of the way in which this issue is becoming more openly discussed, a new web service has been launched at www.mydirectives.com, to let you and those you love and who love you think about and make a record of your wishes, values and preferences. This information will remain on the web and therefore available wherever disaster might strike – Manchester, Madagascar or Melbourne.

5

ACHIEVING WELLBEING

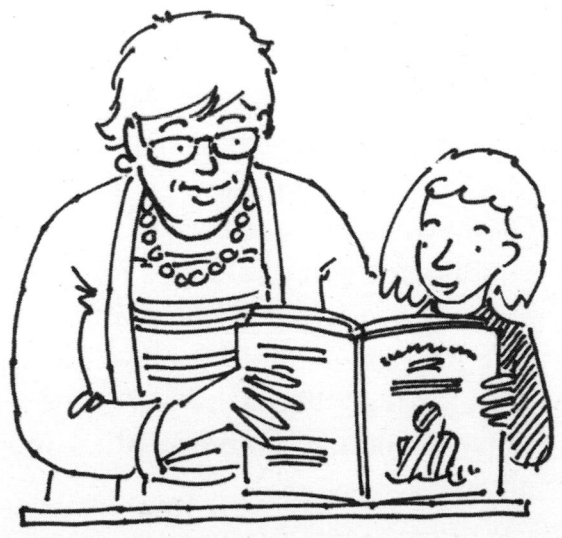

'I am not a number'

People who are 70, just like people at any age, differ from those of the same age in many more ways than they are similar, so generalisations, including those in this book, have to be taken with a pinch of salt. It is true that shared experiences contribute to a common culture – we all remember where we were when we heard of the death of JFK, for example – but we live life as individuals, not as members of groups defined by gender, race or age, and it is important to resist the pressure to conform to the stereotype. In this book, advice has been given about your heart, skin, and lungs. Your aim should be to prevent problems in these organs, to get fitter, to feel – and be – well. But a human being is much more than the sum of all their organs and systems.

Wellbeing is now recognised as a good objective for governments, health services and individuals, even though there is no general agreement about its meaning or measurement. Wellbeing is more than health, because it can include such things as good relationships with neighbours and relatives or sufficient income to take a holiday. Wellbeing, however, is determined by more than your income or your environment: part of it comes from within. People who have a strong religious faith are fortunate because this can contribute to a feeling of wellbeing. Religion is one type of spirituality but there are other sources. Some people are naturally more spiritual, more interested in questions like 'why are we here?' or 'is there a bigger purpose than simply getting through each day without harming other people?' Others are not worried by such questions and just try to lead a fulfilling life, enjoying what they do and making a contribution to others. A number of books tackle these spiritual questions from different points of view.

The books on ageing by the American writer Deepak Chopra would be classified as spiritual by the many people who admire his writing and find his words supportive. His advice to the older generation combines practical advice such as 'spend time with children' with advice many doctors would classify as 'alternative medicine', for example to take a 'teaspoon of ashwagandha (*Withania somnifera*) in warm milk', mixed with advice that some people would consider spiritual, for example, 'release toxic emotions' by practising 'So Hum meditation'.

Two books translated from the French, *Growing Old – A Journey of Self-Discovery* by Danielle Quinodoz and *The Art of Growing Old* by Marie de Hennezel, bring a different approach to spirituality, one that comes not from the Eastern religions but from psychoanalysis. Perhaps this a French way of looking at ageing, because there are cultural differences in the approach to spirituality and ageing. For example, it differs from what many would see as a more practical British approach, as epitomised by Diana Athill's book on ageing and death called *Somewhere Towards the End*.

Her approach is unsentimental and matter of fact. Instead of agonising over the past she says *'Regrets? I say to myself. What regrets? This invisibility may be partly the result of a preponderance of common sense over imagination: regrets are useless, so forget them.'*

Retirement brings problems for some people because they have been defined by their job, by being a teacher, an electrician or a baker, for example, with a clear role that everyone understands. But when this role disappears people may simply start to classify you as 'elderly' and assume, wrongly, that you conform to the stereotype of an 'old person', which is slow, unadventurous and dependent. This is wrong for two reasons: the first being that older people as a group are not slow, unadventurous and dependent; the second reason is that older people differ significantly from one another.

Define yourself or be defined

'No man is an island, entire of itself'
John Donne (1772–1651)

Who we are as individuals is influenced by other people; their expectations, attitudes and prejudices have a bigger influence on us than we like to believe. The expectations of others influence the behaviour of the individual even though that person was never given advice to act in a particular way. Look at what has happened to women over the last fifty years. At first, there were very clear ideas about what jobs should be done by men and what jobs should be done by women, and girls and boys leaving school followed those expectations – girls became nurses or teachers, boys became doctors or engineers. Society has changed, however, partly due to the feminist movement, together with general concern about injustice affecting other excluded groups, such as those from different ethnic groups. Individuals are judged on their merit, not on their gender or race, but there has been no similar mass movement to change the perception of people aged 70, either from the perspective of young people or from the perspective of older people themselves. However, some progress has been made, with discrimination on the basis of age being explicitly identified as unlawful in the Equality Act of 2010. In the United States there has been much more movement, led by organisations like the AARP – the American Association for Retired Persons – Some people have argued this is because retired people in the United States have had to fight much harder and longer than retired people in countries in which pensions and healthcare were made available as a right.

There has never been a golden age for older people, an era in which they were loved and respected. Rich older people were respected as long as they kept the levers of power, but they were not loved for it. The example of King Lear is there for all to see. He held on to power for too long and two of his children turned against him. In the Victorian era, poorer old people often finished up in the workhouse because, even if they were loved, their children with their own large families could not afford to feed their parents as well. Many older people today have financial independence but this has not reduced the tension between the generations. It may, in fact, have increased in the last decade because the 'Baby Boomers' are portrayed as having caused many of the financial and environmental problems of our time.

When you were 36, or 43, nobody had any expectation of what 36-year-olds or 43-year-olds should, or should not, do. You may therefore find it helpful thinking of yourself as being 52 or 48, or some other age for which there are no assumptions. Here are some statements for you to ponder and repeat, at least to yourself:

- I differ from other people aged 70 in many more ways than I resemble them

- I am not really different from the person I was at the age of 54 or 44

- Life has taught me a great deal

- I have a lot to offer other people

- I don't care what other people think about ageing; much of what they believe is wrong

- I know who I am – both my strengths and weaknesses.

These are useful reflections when you are doing your daily exercises! Make up other one-liners about who you are, your uniqueness, and repeat them. This is one way of maintaining a positive view and preventing depression, which affects many people's wellbeing.

STAYING POSITIVE AND DEALING WITH DEPRESSING THOUGHTS

Maintaining your cognitive functions – keeping your brain ticking over – was discussed in chapter 3 on body maintenance. But what about our feelings and emotions – what we feel rather than reason; our mood rather than our memory? How you are feeling – your mood – is influenced more by your relationships with other people than by changes in the brain (although changes in the brain, for example, as a result of a stroke, do have an emotional impact).

The effects of ageing

Depression is a common emotional challenge that faces people aged 70 and upwards. People often say that 'old age is depressing', and simply to point out that it is preferable to the alternative. Death before 70, does not bring a lot of comfort. Some people will need medication for depression and this can be very effective, but for many people the solution is to think differently – take more exercise, and become more engaged with other people. This is not simply a case of saying 'pull yourself together'. It recognises that depressive thoughts are common and serious, sometimes very serious, and that there are both good reasons to be depressed at 70 or 80, and good measures to prevent – and reduce – the problem.

The first step is to try to understand the causes of depression, and those that are more common in older age groups. People of any age can be depressed: by medical problems, by loss of the ability to get out and about, or by poverty. All three reasons are more common as age increases, so some part of the work to help people feel less depressed rests not with the treatment of depression but with effective treatment of medical problems. For example, a hip replacement will be much more effective than anti-depressants for someone who is housebound, lonely and unable to sleep because of pain due to arthritis of the hip joint.

Of course, loneliness is not only the result of becoming housebound because of a disabling disease. For some people loneliness is a consequence of the loss of a partner and the effects of bereavement are still under-estimated by those who have not experienced the devastating effects of the loss of a partner or, particularly distressing, a child. The Charity CRUSE does wonderful work in this area but underfunding continues to prevent some people from benefiting from its services.

The problem of poverty is less easy to tackle because it is rooted in the inequalities that persist in almost every society. Every month people are advised to work longer to build up their pension pot, but this is little comfort to people who are already retired or who are not allowed to work past a fixed age.

There are, however, other causes of depression that are not to do with disease or poverty. These relate to three phases of life – your present position, things that have happened in the past, and things you dread about the future. These are all more significant to someone aged 70 than to someone aged 20.

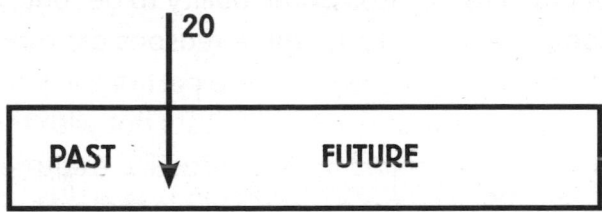

In a developed country the average person aged 20 has experienced very few seriously depressing events; many have never even been to a funeral. At the age of 20, the future is far-reaching and full of opportunity, and although depressing events occur, their effect is often transient. For 70-year-olds, the situation is very different.

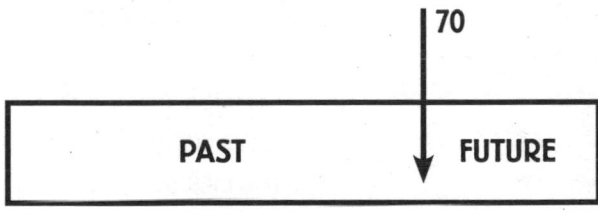

Firstly, many people aged 70 have at least one long-term condition. Some are painless, some have distressing symptoms, but it is natural to feel depressed as the result of developing a disease usually associated with older age, although most people adapt and cope. Secondly, the past is much longer for a 70-year-old and there are usually a number of adverse events that have happened, things that went wrong in life, mistakes that one regrets, and the death of friends, to give three examples. Thirdly, there is the future, now much shorter, and with death as a part of it. For many people, fear about the process of dying is a major cause of anxiety and depression.

Finally, there is the negative image of older people that is commonly held by younger people who dominate the media. The media, particularly television, gets rid of the majority of older presenters and newscasters, particularly older women, thus reinforcing the image of older people as being less attractive and less convincing.

What you can do to minimise depressing thoughts

There are two approaches. The first is to take actions that do not deal directly with how you think and feel

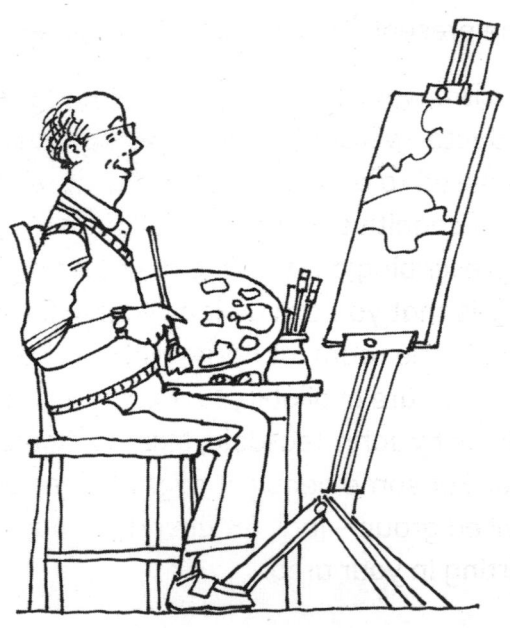

but which have been shown to reduce feelings of depression:

- become more active and increase your physical fitness

- learn a new skill

- get more involved with other people, particularly using your skills to help them.

The second approach is direct and focused on changing your thoughts. The most important step is to spend less time reflecting on and regretting the past and less time worrying about the future. Of course, becoming more active in the ways suggested will also occupy more of your thinking, but the health service is increasingly offering a technique specifically designed to help you focus on the present. This is called 'Mindfulness'.

Mindfulness is a way of thinking more about the present. A doctor will sometimes now refer a person who is depressed to a mindfulness group or to some other form of cognitive or psychological therapy instead of prescribing a drug. One of the strengths of mindfulness is that you can do it by yourself, without a psychologist in the room, at home with the help of one of the CDs which are available, for example, *The Mindful Way Workbook* by John Teasdale, Mark Williams and Zindel Segal. For some people it might be better to start in a supervised group – look for adverts or posters of groups starting in your area.

A mindfulness exercise

Here is what you can try now:

- sit somewhere comfortable but on an upright chair, not a sofa

- concentrate on the weight of your feet on the floor

- listen to your breathing

- look at and concentrate on something still – the view from the window or a picture on the wall

- concentrate on your breathing. Say to yourself 'breathe in' and 'breathe out' ten times

- sit like this for five minutes, aware of your body and surroundings

- if depressing thoughts come into your head, picture them as though they were outside you, like a big advertisement

- repeat the breathing exercise

It sounds simple, but there is already strong evidence from research and the experience of others, that it works. For more information look at www.nhs.uk and search for mindfulness.

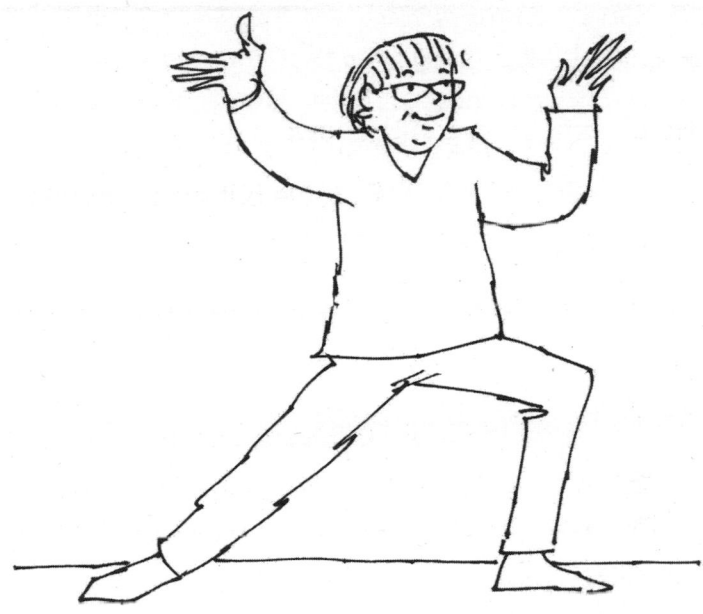

If you can, try Pilates, T'ai Chi, Yoga or the Alexander Technique as well, either online or, better still, in a group. One of them is likely to suit you better than the others. All of these are recommended as being very good for maintaining and improving suppleness, but there is also strong evidence that all forms of exercise are good both for your body and your mind too. In fact, all types of exercise are good for the mind, and actually increase the size of the brain, but these forms of exercise are particularly good because many people find their spiritual dimension and approach helpful. In some ways, they are close to mindfulness and combine the benefits of mindfulness with the benefits of the stretching exercises that we have recommended as part of your daily fitness programme.

177

Depression is common; suicide is thankfully far less common, but it is a possibility that should never be overlooked. If someone says they are thinking of suicide, they should see their doctor without delay. Depression may be common, but it is not inevitable and there is some evidence that older people who do not have to face the challenges of disability or poverty are in fact happier than people in their thirties and forties.

LIVING WELL

Health is much more than the absence of disease. The World Health Organisation has defined health as 'complete physical, social and mental wellbeing' – a state that few people achieve! But the concept of wellness or wellbeing is important, and many people with long-term conditions are nevertheless in a state of wellbeing. On the other hand, there are many younger people who have no disease but who do not seem to be in a state of wellbeing.

Wellbeing is an attitude of mind. Some people appear to be better able to adjust to setbacks and tragedies than others. This is what is called resilience, and probably stems from early childhood, but it is possible to become more resilient by joining groups to learn techniques such as mindfulness. Every day it is good to reflect on the problems and challenges you have already overcome.

Do not regard your seventieth, seventy-third or seventy-eighth birthday as just another birthday: as well as being a cause for celebration, it is a reminder of the need to reflect, think, learn, decide and act to live a full and rewarding life. Thinking is important, but taking action even more so. Some of the action recommended in this book has been physical, not only to get fitter but also for the psychological benefits that result. Some of the actions recommended have been mental, not only to challenge and improve the way your mind works, by learning a new skill for example, but also to make you more resilient, and better able to minimise depressing and negative thinking about the past or the future while increasing your appreciation of the present.

What is increasingly important is to take social action. Retirement comes as a welcome relief to many people, especially those engaged in unsatisfactory or depressing jobs, but even some of them find adjustment to their new life difficult. For people who have had rewarding jobs in which they gained pleasure from using their skills and experience, and respect and positive feedback from the people they were serving, retirement can be a blow. Pre-retirement education, which is offered by many companies, can reduce the adverse effects, but the best approach is to regard retirement as just another change in occupation, albeit one in which your income drops, dramatically for some people. You are starting a new occupation and part of the time should certainly be filled doing the things you have always wanted to do but have not had the time to do when working. It is now clear that working with, and for, the wellbeing of others is very good for you as well as for them.

As was emphasised in the advice on how to improve your memory and reasoning, there is evidence from research that being engaged with other people maintains and improves intellectual functioning. The way it does this is not clear, but it may stem from the need to argue and defend your point of view as well as the need to organise your thoughts. It may also be the interaction with other people that stimulates the mind, and that the increased motivation and morale which results from this improves how you think and how you feel. Here are a few suggestions of what you might want to do:

- work as a volunteer on an issue that you feel strongly about, such as helping people less fortunate than yourself, or protecting the environment. AgeUK is a great organisation and offers a wide range of opportunities (www.ageuk.org.uk). Supporting it and helping it support others will also help you. There are many opportunities for helping people older than yourself, for example, the Silver Sunday initiative launched by the wonderful Joanna Lumley. The aim of Silver Sunday is for more able people to find someone who is unable to get out, and whose children may live far away, and take them out – not just once, although even one trip out can improve wellbeing both through anticipation, and then recollection, of the trip.

- become a member of your local NHS Foundation Trust to contribute your views about current services and future developments of the service in your area (www.foundationtrustwork.org)

- spend more time helping your children and grandchildren, and if your own are far away, help someone else's grandchildren who live near you but whose own grandparents are also far away. Every school needs people to help pupils with reading and arithmetic, and the wisdom that mature volunteers can bring is invaluable.

- work for income, particularly in jobs that younger people do not want to do. There is a new start-up company called Seniors Helping Seniors (www. seniorshelpingseniors.com) which specifically employs people who are older.

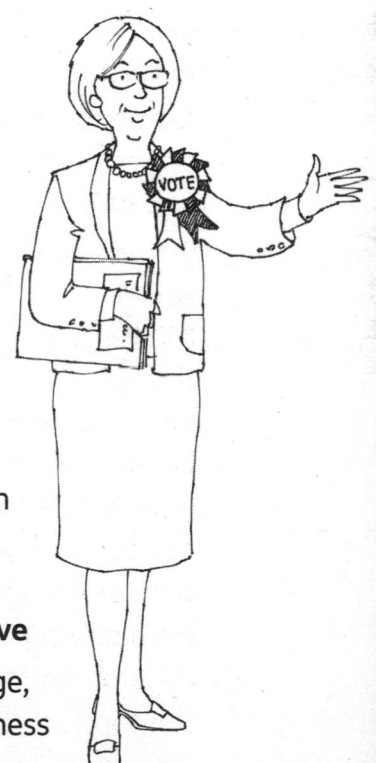

- start a business

- enter politics, run for office in your locality.

New research is much more positive

Much of the negative image of old age, which can affect your feeling of wellness if you believe it too strongly, derives, as we explained earlier, from the results of research that was badly designed – directly comparing people who are 70 or 80 today with people who are 20 today. This is an unfair comparison, of course, because of the advances of diet and healthcare, for example, that make today's environment so much better. In fact, when researchers follow people through life, the rate of decline and loss of function is much less today and and amongst the older generation many abilities have actually improved. Most of the evidence for this is in scientific journals. These can be accessed online at the National Library of Medicine near Washington DC. Put 'healthy ageing' or 'healthy aging' into the search box of www.nlm.nih.gov where over 23,000 scientific articles are presented.

Fortunately, scientists are now writing more for the public – the research on *Our Ageing Brain* is excellently presented for everyone by André Aleman, Professor of Neuropsychology at the University of Gronigen, in his book with that title. Here are some of the book's key positive points, based on the best science and presented with excellent clarity, an unusual combination:

- older people cope better with emotions and stress, and are better at making complex decisions

- some cognitive skills are unaffected by age, or even improve, such as general knowledge and vocabulary

- older people are more stable and can cope better with their feelings

- older people are likely to be nicer than 20 year olds

- wisdom can be defined as having insight into the major issues of life and the ability to make balanced decisions in uncertain situations. We become wiser thanks to the erosion of our mental faculties – the ageing brain works more slowly, and our responses are therefore more sensible.

A major research study of ageing in Europe concluded that to age well the *'continued involvement in physical and social activities'* was important, and recommended that *'far from retiring, engagement with life and society should be the norm for ageing populations'*. Everyone in their seventies has gifts to give. Those gifts are derived from decades of living, from successes and, often more illuminating, mistakes or failures! Looking after others is one of the best ways of looking after yourself. You're 70, don't worry, Sod 70 and go for it!

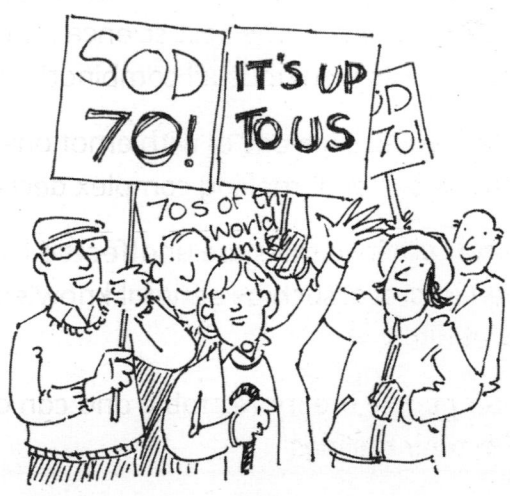

YOUR PROGRAMME FOR WELLBEING

Wellbeing is a difficult concept. Like an elephant, it is easier to recognise than to define, but just as being healthy is more than simply not having disease, so wellbeing is more than being healthy. Wellbeing is a hot topic among economists and many of them would argue that wellbeing is more than happiness because it takes into account practical factors, such as the environment in which you live, and your income. It is difficult to feel a sense of wellbeing if you are constantly in fear of debt.

A summary of the steps you can take to increase your sense of wellbeing:

Get fitter

One of the principal benefits of increasing fitness is not only stronger muscles and more stamina, but the psychological benefit as well, all of which combine to make you feel better.

Be mindful, focus on the present

Mindfulness is a technique designed to help you worry less about the future, and regret less about the past. It is effective even if you only practise for ten minutes a day. This can be done either sitting or walking, or both, and we give advice on the technique on page 176.

Be thankful

In the section on dying well, the techniques that have been found to help people who are seriously or terminally ill include focusing on positive memories and relationships. The same is true for all of us. Focus on the positive at least once or twice a day no matter how bad the day has been. In the words of *Monty Python* 'If life seems jolly rotten, there is always something you've forgotten'.

Help others

For many, helping children and grandchildren is a major source of wellbeing, but with increasing population mobility grandchildren can often live far away. Near you, however, may be other children whose grandparents are distant and who need the type of help that a grandparent would give if they lived nearby. This is just one opportunity for contributing to the wellbeing of others. At the other end of the age range there will be people near you who are older and frailer and in need of help, even if it's just a car ride. Local schools and local branches of Age UK are just two organisations looking for contributions from people with experience.

The Selfish Gene is a book that has attracted worldwide attention. The drive to survive is very important. One of the most successful species on earth is the ant, which appears to demonstrate that there may also be an altruism gene: ants survive by helping one another. Human wellbeing comes from helping others as well as helping oneself.

People in their seventies, as well as society in general, need to recognise that they already give a great deal to the wellbeing of others. Their skills and experience of life could make an even greater contribution to the challenges we all face in the next decade.

FURTHER READING

LEWIS WOLPERT

You're Looking Very Well – The Surprising Nature of Getting Old

Lewis Wolpert is a very distinguished scientist. He also suffered badly from depression and wrote a very clear account not only of his own problem but also of depression in a book called *Malignant Sadness*. In it he describes the response that he has noticed as he has grown older summarised in the comment 'you're looking very well', one often made with a tone of surprise. The book covers a wide range of different topics and has some excellent sections including a very powerful attack, with some relish, on young people who speak negatively about older people:

'Heart-felt perils await people who hold disapproving attitudes about the elderly, a new study suggests. Young and middle-aged adults who endorse negative stereotypes about older people display high rates of strokes, heart attacks and other serious heart problems later in life, compared with ageing peers who view the elderly in generally positive ways. Yale University psychologist Becca Levy found that those who viewed ageing as a positive experience lived an average of seven years longer. This means that a positive image had a greater impact than not smoking or maintaining a healthy weight. Levy says that patronising attitudes and 'elderspeak' – speaking to elders as if they were children – can affect their competence and lifespan. There are claims that optimism and coping styles are more important to successful ageing than physical health.'

DIANA ATHILL

Somewhere Towards The End

At the age of 89, Diane Athill published this memoir of old age. The book is full of descriptions of the benefits she has found from ageing as well, of course, as a honest appreciation of the problems. She has a particularly British, stoical, stiff upper lip approach to life, her no-nonsense approach is clearly illustrated in the quote that follows:

'It seems to me that anyone looking back over eighty-nine years ought to see a landscape pockmarked with regrets. One knows so well, after all, one's own lacks and laziness, omissions, oversights, the innumerable ways in which one falls short of one's own ideals, to say nothing of standards set by other and better people. All this must have thrown up – indeed it certainly did throw up – a large number of regrettable events, yet they have vanished from my sight.

Regrets? I say to myself. What regrets? This invisibility may be partly the result of a preponderance of common sense over imagination: regrets are useless, so forget them.'

DANIELLE QINODOZ

Growing Old – The Journey of Self Discovery

This book is written by a psychoanalyst. Qinodoz is from the French part of Switzerland so, culturally, probably identifies more with France than with Germany. From a psychoanalytic perspective, growing old is a journey of self-discovery. She reflects on the problems that the psychoanalyst faces in growing old. One would expect a psychoanalyst to encourage people to reflect the depth of the past, but she also gives some very practical advice on focusing on the present:

'The present is free and distinct from the past ... All of this is a matter of personal creativity; those who can keep hold of the qualities of their childhood as they grow old are very much at an advantage in this respect. The present is free and distinct from the future. Maintaining the freedom of the present also implies preventing it from being disrupted by the future.'

MARIE DE HENNEZEL

The Art of Growing Old – Aging with Grace

It is fair to say that British people and French people have a different culture. French people undoubtedly value intellectual discussion whereas the British approach may be regarded as more practical and down to earth. Diana Athill's memoir *Somewhere Towards The End* is very clear and direct. Marie de Hennezel, a French therapist, has written a different type of book, more discursive and reflective. She focuses on fears about old age and has many fascinating interviews, in particular with 'remarkable elderly people' and from this there are sections in the book such as 'keys to a happy old age' with an important chapter on 'knowing how to die':

'Instead of confronting this fear, we ward it off by clinging to our youth in a rather pathetic state of denial. In so doing, we run the risk of missing out on what I call here "the work of growing old" – that is to say, cultivating a positive awareness of ageing. If you are not prepared for growing old, if you have not developed the necessary inner resources for getting through this last stage of life, you risk going through hell.'

ANDRÉ ALEMAN

Our Ageing Brain – How Our Mental Capacities Develop as We Grow Older

André Aleman is Professor of Cognitive Neuropsychology at the University of Groningen in the Netherlands. Essentially a science book, Aleman's work would be an excellent read for doctors in training as well as members of the public. His insights are very encouraging and counter many of the established beliefs about intellectual decline in old age. Based solely on scientific evidence, he says that 'a positive attitude to ageing has a greater impact on health than physical health, smoking or obesity'. Aleman reminds us that speed is not everything, and that the wisdom of age comes from the very fact that we do not jump quickly to conclusions. He also emphasises the importance of exercise, like T'ai Chi for example, that brings together the physical, psychological and social aspects of growing old. The book ends with the following comforting observation:

'Spiritually, religion and mindfulness have a proven positive influence on mental health.'

DEEPAK CHOPRA

Ageless Body, Timeless Mind

Dr Deepak Chopra is the founder of the Chopra Centre for Wellbeing in Carlsbad, California. His books include titles such as *Perfect Health, Boundless Energy, Perfect Digestion* and, a very welcome addition, *Golf for Enlightenment.*

There is no doubt that he has been strongly influenced by Eastern religions and in many ways the book has all the resonance of California in the 1960s with people thinking in new ways about our life and existence. There are, however, many practical statements and pieces of advice in the book. He also provides useful lists, for example, the ten new assumptions with number ten being 'we are not victims of aging, sickness and death, which are part of the scenery'. The book also contains lots of practical information, for example, on longevity and weight, and longevity and exercise. The book has a very stimulating combination of spiritual statements such as 'the mind and body are inseparably one' and practical information such as 'thirty minutes of dancing burns the same amount of calories as twenty minutes of tennis or twenty-five minutes of mowing the lawn'. Here is an example of both his writing and what he would probably regard as the core message of the book:

'Life is a creative enterprise. There are many levels of creation and therefore many levels of possible mastery. To completely loving, non-judgemental, and self-accepting is an exalted goal, but the important thing is to work from a concept of wholeness. Because society lacks a vision of the road's end, the eminent psychiatrist Erik Erikson laments, "Our civilization does not really harbour a concept of the whole of life." The new paradigm provides us with such a concept, knitting body, mind, and spirit into a unity. The later years should be a time when life becomes whole. The circle closes and life's purpose is fulfilled. In that regard, active mastery is not just a way to survive to extreme old age – it is the road to freedom.'

VIRGINA IRONSIDE

The Virginia Monologues – Why Growing Old is Great

Virginia Ironside is a famous agony aunt in the UK. She writes well and responds clearly to the questions raised. This book was stimulated by her sixtieth birthday. It is amusing and instructive. She writes about memory, confidence, death, sex and wisdom. There is lots of practical advice hidden within this dialogue prose and this would make a very good present for someone's sixtieth or seventieth birthday, particularly for a woman. Here is her bottom line:

'In the run-up to my sixtieth birthday I found that I, too, was starting to get brainwashed into thinking that "old" was something ghastly, something to be avoided at all costs. It was only when the day actually came that I started to realise that being old isn't something to deny or hush up or apologize for. Far from it. It's something to celebrate.'

ATUL GAWNDE

Being Mortal; Illness, Medicine and What Matters in the End

Atul Gawande is a surgeon who writes excellently about medicine and healthcare, principally about how clinical practice can be made better and safer. In this book he tackles an issue that is a growing concern – over-treatment. In an era in which every country is under pressure to put more resources into healthcare, there is a parallel campaign to reduce both over-treatment and over-diagnosis. Over-diagnosis results from many different factors, from the development of new tests, from the increasing range of diagnostic technology in labs and imaging departments and from the enthusiasm of doctors who want to tackle disease earlier, for example, by creating a new entity called pre-diabetes. This same enthusiasm, made with the best of intentions, also leads to over-treatment particularly at the end of life. And it is Atul Gawnde's clinical experience combined with the story of his father's final illness that forms the central core of this fascinating book:

'Being mortal is about the struggle to cope with the constraints of our biology, with the limits set by genes and cells and flesh and bone. Medical science has given us remarkable power to push against these limits, and the potential value of this power was a central reason I became a doctor. But, again and again, I have seen the damage we in medicine do when we fail to acknowledge that such power is finite and always will be.'

INDEX

psychological fitness 51
pulse 18, 91, 92

reasoning abilities 64, 67–8
religious beliefs 160, 166, 191
resilience 178, 179
resistance (exercise) bands
29–30, 40–1, 53
retirement 69, 168, 179
rheumatoid arthritis 105

scientific studies of ageing
181–3
sedentary lifestyle 16, 25, 78,
95
sexual health maintenance
113–16
shingles 149
shoulder exercises 32, 36, 37
skin cancer 129, 130
skin maintenance 127–30
sleep, good 65–6
smoking 8, 59–60, 85–6, 87–90,
91, 101
spine maintenance 106–10
spirituality 160–1, 166–8, 177,
191
stair climbing 20–1, 24
stamina 18, 19, 20–8, 24, 87
statins 92, 96
stiffness 105
stooping 27, 106, 108, 109
strength training 18, 19, 29–30,
53, 96, 99
stretching exercises 36–47,
108–9, 177
stroke 18, 78, 150, 171
FAST checklist 61–2

suicidal thoughts 178
sun safety 128–9
suppleness 18, 19, 32–3, 36,
45, 103–4, 105, 177
surgical operations 88, 105,
137–8
swimming 22, 24, 86

T'ai Chi 101, 177, 191
teeth grinding 126
testosterone 96, 114, 115
thyroid disorders 84
tinnitus 133
tooth and gum maintenance
123–7

ulcerative colitis 75
ulcers 112, 126, 130
uniqueness, personal 170–1
upper limb exercises 36, 38–41

vaccinations 86, 147–9
vision maintenance 130–2
vitamin D 99, 100, 102, 129
volunteering 68–9, 70, 180

walking 22, 23, 24, 25–8, 51,
52, 60, 78, 80, 81, 99, 155
waterworks maintenance
117–22
weight loss, unplanned 84
weight management 60,
79–81, 83, 111
wellbeing 166–86
wisdom 183, 191
wrinkles 128

yoga 177

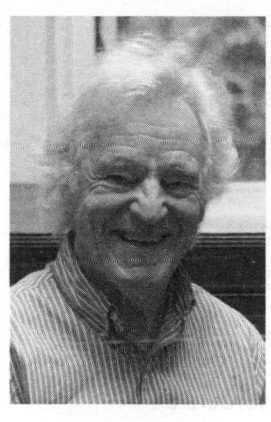

ABOUT THE AUTHOR

Muir Gray has worked in public health for over 40 years. Having qualified in medicine in his home town of Glasgow, he worked in hospitals in Glasgow and Aberdeen before entering the Public Health Service in 1972 to take up a job in the City of Oxford Health Dept.

The first phase of his career focused on disease prevention, particularly helping people stop smoking, and population ageing. His work with older people focused not only on keeping healthy through the promotion of exercise but also on issues such as preventing hypothermia by better housing. In this period he wrote and edited the books *Care for Elderly People in General Practice* and *Prevention of Disease in the Elderly*. Muir went on to develop screening programmes in the NHS for pregnant women, children, adults and older people. This included offering men aged sixty-five screening for abdominal aortic aneurysm and, for both men and women, screening for colorectal cancer.

Muir helped develop the National Library for Health, was founder of the National Knowledge Services and was integral in developing NHS Choices (www.nhs.uk), which now has over 40 million visits a month.

He was the Chief Knowledge Officer of the NHS and received first a CBE and then seven years later a Knighthood for services to the NHS.

Muir is now working with NHS England and Public Health England to bring about a transformation of care with the aim of increasing value. Instead of thinking about health centres and hospitals being like supermarkets, offering all things to all people, his company Better Value Healthcare is developing integrated care focused on people with a common need, such as people with heart disease or people at the end of life. This new approach to healthcare also requires the service to focus on the needs of patients and their carers, based on the knowledge that self-care and informal care by relatives and volunteers are the principal types of care, even for people who are very disabled.

Muir is also founder of the charity the National Campaign for Walking, which promotes walking for health, and you can see him promoting walking on Youtube. He has set up a second charity to contribute to the struggle against climate change by helping the NHS reduce its carbon footprint. He has also published a short summary of the scientific evidence on which this book is based called *An Antidote To Ageing*.